OBSERVATIC
IN A LEARNING

MW01063063

Workshop Summary

Claudia Grossmann and Joe Alper, *Rapporteurs*

A Learning Health System Activity

Roundtable on Value & Science-Driven Health Care

INSTITUTE OF MEDICINE
OF THE NATIONAL ACADEMIES

THE NATIONAL ACADEMIES PRESS
Washington, D.C.
www.nap.edu

THE NATIONAL ACADEMIES PRESS   500 Fifth Street, NW   Washington, DC 20001

NOTICE: The workshop that is the subject of this workshop summary was approved by the Governing Board of the National Research Council, whose members are drawn from the councils of the National Academy of Sciences, the National Academy of Engineering, and the Institute of Medicine.

This activity was supported by an unnumbered agreement between the National Academy of Sciences and the Patient-Centered Outcomes Research Institute. The views presented in this publication do not necessarily reflect the views of the organizations or agencies that provided support for the activity.

International Standard Book Number-13:   978-0-309-29081-4
International Standard Book Number-10:   0-309-29081-3

Additional copies of this workshop summary are available for sale from the National Academies Press, 500 Fifth Street, NW, Keck 360, Washington, DC 20001; (800) 624-6242 or (202) 334-3313; http://www.nap.edu.

For more information about the Institute of Medicine, visit the IOM home page at: www.iom.edu.

The serpent has been a symbol of long life, healing, and knowledge among almost all cultures and religions since the beginning of recorded history. The serpent adopted as a logotype by the Institute of Medicine is a relief carving from ancient Greece, now held by the Staatliche Museen in Berlin.

Suggested citation: IOM (Institute of Medicine). 2013. *Observational studies in a learning health system: Workshop summary.* Washington, DC: The National Academies Press.

"Knowing is not enough; we must apply. Willing is not enough; we must do."

—Goethe

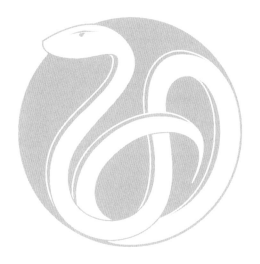

INSTITUTE OF MEDICINE
OF THE NATIONAL ACADEMIES

Advising the Nation. Improving Health.

THE NATIONAL ACADEMIES
Advisers to the Nation on Science, Engineering, and Medicine

The **National Academy of Sciences** is a private, nonprofit, self-perpetuating society of distinguished scholars engaged in scientific and engineering research, dedicated to the furtherance of science and technology and to their use for the general welfare. Upon the authority of the charter granted to it by the Congress in 1863, the Academy has a mandate that requires it to advise the federal government on scientific and technical matters. Dr. Ralph J. Cicerone is president of the National Academy of Sciences.

The **National Academy of Engineering** was established in 1964, under the charter of the National Academy of Sciences, as a parallel organization of outstanding engineers. It is autonomous in its administration and in the selection of its members, sharing with the National Academy of Sciences the responsibility for advising the federal government. The National Academy of Engineering also sponsors engineering programs aimed at meeting national needs, encourages education and research, and recognizes the superior achievements of engineers. Dr. C. D. Mote, Jr., is president of the National Academy of Engineering.

The **Institute of Medicine** was established in 1970 by the National Academy of Sciences to secure the services of eminent members of appropriate professions in the examination of policy matters pertaining to the health of the public. The Institute acts under the responsibility given to the National Academy of Sciences by its congressional charter to be an adviser to the federal government and, upon its own initiative, to identify issues of medical care, research, and education. Dr. Harvey V. Fineberg is president of the Institute of Medicine.

The **National Research Council** was organized by the National Academy of Sciences in 1916 to associate the broad community of science and technology with the Academy's purposes of furthering knowledge and advising the federal government. Functioning in accordance with general policies determined by the Academy, the Council has become the principal operating agency of both the National Academy of Sciences and the National Academy of Engineering in providing services to the government, the public, and the scientific and engineering communities. The Council is administered jointly by both Academies and the Institute of Medicine. Dr. Ralph J. Cicerone and Dr. C. D. Mote, Jr., are chair and vice chair, respectively, of the National Research Council.

www.national-academies.org

PLANNING COMMITTEE ON OBSERVATIONAL STUDIES IN A LEARNING HEALTH SYSTEM[1]

RALPH I. HORWITZ (*Co-Chair*), Senior Vice President, Clinical Sciences Evaluation, GlaxoSmithKline

JOE V. SELBY (*Co-Chair*), Executive Director, Patient-Centered Outcomes Research Institute

ANIRBAN BASU, Associate Professor and Director, Health Economics and Outcomes Methodology, University of Washington

TROYEN A. BRENNAN, Executive Vice President and Chief Medical Officer, CVS/Caremark

STEVEN N. GOODMAN, Associate Dean for Clinical & Translational Research, Stanford University School of Medicine, Stanford University

LOUIS B. JACQUES, Director, Coverage and Analysis Group, Centers for Medicare & Medicaid Services

JEROME P. KASSIRER, Distinguished Professor, Tufts University School of Medicine

MICHAEL S. LAUER, Director, Division of Cardiovascular Sciences, National Heart, Lung, and Blood Institute

DAVID MADIGAN, Chair of Statistics, Columbia University

SHARON-LISE T. NORMAND, Professor, Department of Biostatistics and Health Care Policy, Harvard University

RICHARD PLATT, Chair of Ambulatory Care and Prevention and Chair of Population Medicine, Harvard Pilgrim Health Care Institute

BURTON H. SINGER, Professor, Emerging Pathogens Institute, University of Florida

JEAN R. SLUTSKY, Director, Center for Outcomes and Evidence, Agency for Healthcare Research and Quality

ROBERT TEMPLE, Deputy Director for Clinical Science, Center for Drug Evaluation and Research, U.S. Food and Drug Administration

IOM Staff

KATHERINE BURNS, Program Assistant
CLAUDIA GROSSMANN, Senior Program Officer
DIEDTRA HENDERSON, Program Officer
ELIZABETH JOHNSTON, Program Assistant
ELIZABETH ROBINSON, Research Associate
VALERIE ROHRBACH, Senior Program Assistant

---

[1] Institute of Medicine planning committees are solely responsible for organizing the workshop, identifying topics, and choosing speakers. The responsibility for the published workshop summary rests with the workshop rapporteurs and the institution.

ROUNDTABLE ON VALUE & SCIENCE-DRIVEN HEALTH CARE[1]

---

[1] Institute of Medicine forums and roundtables do not issue, review, or approve individual documents. The responsibility for the published workshop summary rests with the workshop rapporteurs and the institution.

Institute of Medicine
Roundtable on Value & Science-Driven Health Care
Charter and Vision Statement

Vision: Our vision is for the development of a continuously learning health system in which science, informatics, incentives, and culture are aligned for continuous improvement and innovation, with best practices seamlessly embedded in the care process, patients and families active participants in all elements, and new knowledge captured as an integral by-product of the care experience.

Goal: By the year 2020, 90 percent of clinical decisions will be supported by accurate, timely, and up-to-date clinical information and will reflect the best available evidence. We believe that this presents a tangible focus for progress toward our vision, that Americans ought to expect at least this level of performance, that it should be feasible with existing resources and emerging tools, and that measures can be developed to track and stimulate progress.

Context: As unprecedented developments in the diagnosis, treatment, and long-term management of disease bring Americans closer than ever to the promise of personalized health care, we are faced with similarly unprecedented challenges to identify and deliver the care most appropriate for individual needs and conditions. Care that is important is often not delivered. Care that is delivered is often not important. In part, this is due to our failure to apply the evidence that we have about the medical care that is most effective—a failure related to shortfalls in provider knowledge and accountability, inadequate care coordination and support, lack of insurance, poorly aligned payment incentives, and misplaced patient expectations. Increasingly, it is also a result of our limited capacity for timely generation of evidence on the relative effectiveness, efficiency, and safety of available and emerging interventions. Improving the value of the return on our health care investment is a vital imperative that will require much greater capacity to evaluate high-priority clinical interventions, stronger links between clinical research and practice, and reorientation of the incentives to apply new insights. We must quicken our efforts to position evidence development and application as natural outgrowths of clinical care to foster health care that learns.

Approach: The Institute of Medicine Roundtable on Value & Science-Driven Health Care serves as a forum to facilitate the collaborative assessment and action around issues central to achieving the vision and goal stated. The challenges are myriad and include issues that must be addressed to improve evidence development, evidence application, and the capacity to advance progress on both dimensions. To address these challenges, as leaders in their fields, Roundtable members work with their colleagues to identify the issues not being adequately addressed, the nature of the barriers and possible solutions, and the priorities for action and marshal the resources of the sectors represented on the Roundtable to work for sustained public-private cooperation for change. Activities include collaborative exploration of new and expedited approaches to assessing the effectiveness of diagnostic and treatment interventions, better use of the patient care experience to generate evidence on the effectiveness and efficiency of care, identification of assessment priorities, and communication strategies to enhance provider and patient understanding and support for interventions proven to work best and deliver value in health care.

Core concepts and principles: For the purpose of the Roundtable activities, we define science-driven health care broadly to mean that, to the greatest extent possible, the decisions that shape the health and health care of Americans—by patients, providers, payers, and policy makers alike—will be grounded in a reliable evidence base, will account appropriately for individual variation in patient needs, and will support the generation of new insights on clinical effectiveness. Evidence is generally considered to be information from clinical experience that has met some established test of validity, and the appropriate standard is determined according to the requirements of the intervention and clinical circumstance. Processes that involve the development and use of evidence should be accessible and transparent to all stakeholders.

A common commitment to certain principles and priorities guides the activities of the Roundtable and its members, including the commitment to the right health care for each person; putting the best evidence into practice; establishing the effectiveness, efficiency, and safety of the medical care delivered; building constant measurement into our health care investments; the establishment of health care data as a public good; shared responsibility distributed equitably across stakeholders, both public and private; collaborative stakeholder involvement in priority settings; transparency in the execution of activities and reporting of results; and subjugation of individual political or stakeholder perspectives in favor of the common good.

Reviewers

This workshop summary has been reviewed in draft form by individuals chosen for their diverse perspectives and technical expertise, in accordance with procedures approved by the National Research Council's Report Review Committee. The purpose of this independent review is to provide candid and critical comments that will assist the institution in making its published workshop summary as sound as possible and to ensure that the workshop summary meets institutional standards for objectivity, evidence, and responsiveness to the study charge. The review comments and draft manuscript remain confidential to protect the integrity of the process. We wish to thank the following individuals for their review of this workshop summary:

John Concato, U.S. Department of Veterans Affairs
Sheldon Greenfield, University of California, Irvine
Harold Sox, Dartmouth Geisel School of Medicine
Alexander Walker, Harvard School of Public Health

Although the reviewers listed above have provided many constructive comments and suggestions, they did not see the final draft of the workshop summary before its release. The review of this workshop summary was overseen by **Eric Larson,** Group Health Research Institute. Appointed by the Institute of Medicine, he was responsible for making certain that an independent examination of this workshop summary was carried out in accordance with institutional procedures and that all review comments were carefully considered. Responsibility for the final content of this workshop summary rests entirely with the rapporteurs and the institution.

Foreword

Clinical research strains to keep up with the rapid and iterative evolution of medical interventions, clinical practice innovation, and the increasing demand for information on the clinical effectiveness of these advancements. Given the growing availability of archived and real-time digital health data and the opportunities this data provides for research, as well as the increasing number of studies using prospectively collected clinical data, the Institute of Medicine's (IOM's) Roundtable on Value & Science-Driven Health Care, with the support of the Patient-Centered Outcomes Research Institute (PCORI), convened a workshop on Observational Studies in a Learning Health System, which is summarized in this publication. Participants included experts from a wide range of disciplines—clinical researchers, statisticians, biostatisticians, epidemiologists, health care informaticians, health care analytics, research funders, health products industry, clinicians, payers, and regulators.

The workshop explored leading edge approaches to observational studies, charted a course for the use of the growing health data utility, and identified opportunities to advance progress. This publication summarizes discussions that considered concepts of rigorous observational study design and analysis, emerging statistical methods, opportunities and challenges of observational studies to complement evidence from experimental methods, treatment heterogeneity, and effectiveness estimates tailored toward individual patients.

The work of the Roundtable is focused on moving toward a continuously learning health system, one where every health care encounter is an opportunity for learning and evidence is applied to ensure and improve best care practices. Since its inception in 2006, the Roundtable has set out to help realize this vision through the involvement and support of senior leadership from key health care stakeholders. In engaging the nation's leaders in workshops and other activities, Roundtable members and colleagues contribute to progress on issues important to advancing the development and use of a digital health data utility for knowledge generation and continuous improvement.

Building on this groundwork, the objectives of this workshop were to explore the role of observational studies in the generation of evidence to guide clinical and health policy decisions. Issues of rigor, internal validity and bias were engaged, as well as opportunities for using observational studies to generalize findings from randomized controlled trials (RCTs), and to better understand treatment heterogeneity. Workshop speakers and individual participants strove to identify stakeholder needs and barriers to the broader application of observational studies-generated evidence for decision making by engaging colleagues from disciplines typically underrepresented in clinical evidence discussions.

A number of specific issues were identified by speakers and participants who spoke in the course of the workshop as especially important to accelerate progress in the appropriate use of observational studies for evidence generation. In the following sections we highlight some of the key points that emerged from each of the four topics in the workshop.

The first theme covered in the workshop focused on the challenge to mitigate the potential effects of bias in the absence of randomization. Two of the speakers, Small and Basu, emphasized the role of instrumental variables (IVs) as "natural randomizers" to achieve similarity between compared groups that would strengthen causal inferences. Their contributions included a list of examples of potential IVs, including distance to hospital or health care provider, timing of hospital admission, and insurance plan coverage, among others. The current lack of efficient IVs was noted by several individual workshop participants to be a major limitation of the method. A presentation from Ryan of the Observational Medical Outcomes Partnership discussed an empirical approach to measuring bias and error in observational research. Their findings that bias is common and differential by design, analysis, source of data and outcome definition was accompanied by straightforward strategies to measure and mitigate the effects of bias.

Heterogeneity of treatment effect (HTE) was the second theme of the workshop and was discussed both in theory and in specific examples. The lack of frequent HTE in the analysis of many RCTs led some participants to wonder how much HTE is present in clinical research. This view was challenged by Kent who attributed the lack of reliably measured HTE to the failure of information and the low analytical power of conventional analytic methods. It was also noted that many "traditional" RCTs use exclusion and inclusion criteria that may remove HTE from the study. This point was illustrated by one example, presented by Hlatky that described HTE in a comparative effectiveness study of coronary artery bypass grafting and percutaneous coronary intervention using a 20 percent sample of Medicare data.

The third topic engaged by the workshop was generalizing RCT results to broader populations. A presentation by Hernán shifted the emphasis of discussion from the validity of the answer (bias reduction) to emphasize the quality of the question. One of the points highlighted by this discussion was how central the research question is to issues in methods, analysis, and inferences from clinical research. A resulting suggestion, made by individual workshop participants who spoke, was that the analysis of observational studies and RCTs be the same, except for adjustment for any potential baseline confounding.

The final session was on individual risk prediction. The sentiment expressed by many workshop participants was captured in one of the talks that titled its first slide: "When the average applies to no one." Speakers took on the pragmatic issues of prediction, including the observation that most risk prediction tools do not tailor the instrument to reflect the variability among patients in age, comorbidities, extent and severity of disease, or other relevant features. Among the hopeful suggestions that arose from this session was that electronic health records may be useful to build prediction models, but this was balanced by the acknowledgment that incomplete patient follow up remains the largest barrier to creating prediction rules that are helpful to patients and physicians. Tatonetti presented a data-driven prediction of drug effects and interactions using observational data and addressing "synthetic" associations that occurred when drugs that are co-prescribed are also associated with the adverse risks of the other medicine. The authors described a new method, the Statistical Correction of Uncharacterized Bias, to minimize these synthetic associations and validated the method by returning to the laboratory for experimental confirmation of drug disease interactions.

Multiple individuals donated valuable time toward the development of this publication. *We would like to acknowledge and offer strong appreciation for the contributors to this volume for their presence at the workshop and their efforts to further develop their presentations into the summaries contained in this publication.* We are especially indebted to those who provided sterling expert guidance as members of the Planning Committee: Anirban Basu (University of Washington), Troyen Brennan (CVS/Caremark), Steven Goodman (Stanford University), Louis Jacques (Centers for Medicare & Medicaid Services), Jerome Kassirer (Tufts University School of Medicine), Michael Lauer (National Heart, Lung, and Blood Institute), David Madigan (Columbia University), Sharon-Lise

Normand (Harvard University), Richard Platt (Harvard Pilgrim Health Care Institute), Burton Singer (University of Florida), Jean Slutsky (Agency for Healthcare Research and Quality), and Robert Temple (U.S. Food and Drug Administration).

Various IOM Roundtable staff played instrumental roles in coordinating the workshop and translating the workshop proceedings into this summary, including Claudia Grossmann, Elizabeth Johnston, Valerie Rohrbach, Julia Sanders, Rob Saunders, and Barret Zimmermann. We would like to recognize Joe Alper for his assistance in drafting this publication. Finally, we want to thank Daniel Bethea, Marton Cavani, Laura Harbold DeStefano, and Chelsea Frakes for helping to coordinate various aspects of review, production, and publication.

An effective and efficient health care system requires a continually evolving evidence base to guide clinical decisions at the patient level and policy decisions at the level of the population level. Observational studies play an important role in complementing other research methods and building this evidence base. We believe *Observational Studies in a Learning Health System: Workshop Summary* will be a valuable resource as efforts to ensure that learning from digital health data are a crucial part of any health system.

Ralph Horwitz, Co-*Chair*
Planning Committee on Observational Studies in a
Learning Health System
Senior Vice President, Clinical Sciences Evaluation
GlaxoSmithKline

Joe Selby, Co-*Chair*
Planning Committee on Observational Studies in a
Learning Health System
Executive Director
Patient-Centered Outcomes Research Institute

J. Michael McGinnis
Executive Director, Roundtable on
Value & Science-Driven Health Care
Institute of Medicine

Contents

Acronyms and Abbreviations

AHRQ   Agency for Healthcare Research and Quality

CABG   coronary artery bypass grafting
CMS   Centers for Medicare & Medicaid Services
Csxover   case-crossover study

EHR   electronic health record

FDA   U.S. Food and Drug Administration

IOM   Institute of Medicine
IPSM   implicit propensity score matching
ITT   intent to treat analysis
IV   instrumental variable

OMOP   Observational Medical Outcomes Partnership

PCI   percutaneous coronary intervention
PCORI   Patient-Centered Outcomes Research Institute
PSA   prostate-specific antigen

RCT   randomized controlled (clinical) trial

SCCS   self-controlled case series

1

Introduction[1]

Clinical research is changing, although perhaps not fast enough to meet the challenges and seize the opportunities presented. The constantly increasing diversity and sophistication of health care interventions hold great promise to provide gains in health but also raise substantial challenges to the pace and nature of research on the effectiveness of treatments. New tools are also emerging, however. These tools have the potential to accelerate the research process and to tailor it more to the question being asked, to allow, in effect, a diverse, portfolio-based approach to clinical research that applies the most appropriate methods, given the specific requirements of the situation. This approach includes the conduct of randomized controlled trials (RCTs) as well as the leveraging of the information collected in the process of delivering care through observational studies to drive processes for continuous improvement, which is at the heart of a learning health system.

All research methods have advantages and disadvantages; therefore, the role of specific methods in contributing to a learning health system varies according to the framing of the questions being asked and the context in which the research is being carried out. Although RCTs have strong internal validity, their use of well-defined test and control populations limits their applicability to patients in the real world, who often have characteristics

---

[1] The planning committee's role was limited to planning the workshop, and the workshop summary has been prepared by the workshop rapporteurs as a factual summary of what occurred at the workshop. Statements, recommendations, and opinions expressed are those of individual presenters and participants and are not necessarily endorsed or verified by the Institute of Medicine, and they should not be construed as reflecting any group consensus.

such as comorbidities that would disqualify them from most RCTs. In addition, because of their extended timelines and costs, which can run in the range of $300 million to $600 million (IOM, 2009), RCTs are an impractical approach to address many important questions.

Observational studies face issues of bias, but when they are used correctly, they can provide information on the effectiveness of therapies in real-world clinical practice. Observational studies can detect signals about the benefits and risks of various therapies in the general population, identify rare side effects and benefits that are beyond the reach of RCTs, and provide community-level data that can lead to new hypotheses that can then be tested in clinical trials. In addition, observational studies can be used in conjunction with RCTs to test the external validity of the RCTs by expanding the clinical settings to a more representative population and to assess the heterogeneity of the treatment response. These approaches will not replace RCTs but can complement them in building the body of evidence on which health decisions can be made.

Today, the most rapidly growing resource for scientific progress in health and health care is the nation's clinical data infrastructure. The increased adoption of electronic health records, with 44 percent of hospitals and 40 percent of physicians' offices having at least a basic system (Robert Wood Johnson Foundation, 2013), and the proliferation of mobile sensors and devices, such as the FitBit activity tracker and wireless-enabled scales, have created a wealth of health data that can serve as a resource for learning. This resource, which can be thought of as a new form of public utility, coupled with advances in scientific and statistical methods, makes an examination of the role of observational studies in a learning health system timely.

The purpose of the workshop described here was to identify the leading approaches to observational studies, chart the course for the use of this growing utility, and guide and grow their use in the most responsible fashion possible.

THE ROLE OF OBSERVATIONAL STUDIES
IN A LEARNING HEALTH SYSTEM

An effective and efficient health care system requires a continually evolving evidence base to guide clinical decisions at the patient level and policy decisions at the level of the population. To meet this need, the methods used must be rigorous and the evidence must be valid and generalizable. Approaches to generating the kind of evidence needed to guide decisions will vary on the basis of the question asked, access to data or research subjects, the availability of resources, and the ultimate use of the results. When the evidence needs of the health system as a whole are considered, the need for a diversity of approaches to match the wide array of situations and needs is clear.

Clinical research methods can be differentiated in several different ways, with the most fundamental differentiator being whether an approach is observational or experimental. This distinction is defined primarily by whether randomization is employed. Randomization can confer protection from certain biases but can involve logistical and even ethical challenges. Methods that do not employ randomization and that rely on data collected as part of other processes, such as the delivery of care, face analytical challenges but are theoretically easier to carry out and are more likely to produce results that are representative of the environment in which they are being used to inform decision making.

Given this differentiation, several challenges and opportunities are associated with the use of observational studies to generate evidence and inform decision making. The challenges include biases related to the measurement methods used, the population selected for study, the time available for the study, and confounding by medical indication. Because interventions are not randomly assigned in observational studies and the study environment is not tightly controlled, causal relationships are harder to draw. However, innovations in statistical methods, such as instrumental variable (IV) and propensity scores, have allowed progress in addressing these challenges to be made. Data quality, in particular, for studies done with data not collected for research purposes, is an additional challenge.

Observational studies also provide opportunities for clinical research. They require fewer resources and in some cases require the collection of minimal to no additional data beyond those that are routinely collected, and they can often be done more expeditiously than clinical trials. Because observational studies require minimal modification of routine processes, they can provide insight into real-world processes and effects that may more closely mirror those in the decision-making environment in which their results are used. In addition, the broader inclusiveness of observational studies means that the population studied is more likely to mirror the population of patients whose care their findings can inform.

One area of promise for observational studies is provision of a better understanding of heterogeneity in the responses to treatment and the effects of treatment. Although attempts to obtain an understanding of this heterogeneity were made through the analysis of subgroups of individuals participating in RCTs, the size of observational studies provides a greater power to detect and understand heterogeneity among subsets of a larger study population. Finally, data collected in the context of routine care or for observational studies can be used to develop predictive models to, for example, help clinicians and patients make health care decisions on the basis of data from patients who are the most like the patients being treated.

THE ROUNDTABLE AND THE *LEARNING HEALTH SYSTEM* SERIES

Since its founding at the Institute of Medicine in 2006, the Roundtable on Value & Science-Driven Health Care has brought together leaders from throughout the health system to accelerate the development of a continuously learning health system. A learning health system is one in which science, informatics, incentives, and the culture of the health care system are aligned to create a continuous learning loop. In a learning health care system, evidence and best practices are embedded in health and health care services and new knowledge is routinely captured as a by-product from each interaction with the system (see Figure 1-1). To achieve this ambitious goal, the Roundtable convenes meetings of key leaders in health care, holds public workshops, stewards collaborative projects that advance a learning system, and authors reports and related publications.

During the past 7 years, the Roundtable has produced 14 publications, including this one, in its *Learning Health System* series. The topics covered

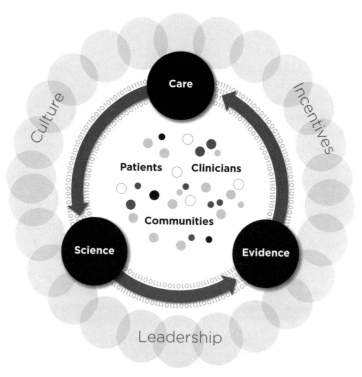

FIGURE 1-1 Schematic of a learning health system.
SOURCE: IOM, 2012.

in these publications span a number of the elements necessary for transformation of the system, including clinical research, the digital infrastructure, engaging patients and the public, focusing on value and financial incentives, and applying lessons from other industries to health and health care. The publications have explored stakeholder perspectives on each issue and have identified priorities for advancement and areas in need of collaborative action.

Another vehicle for the Roundtable's work is a series of Innovation Collaboratives in which key leaders in health and health care participate in collaborative activities that advance the science and increase the value of the health system. The Innovation Collaboratives currently focus on six overlapping and complementary areas: clinical effectiveness research, digital infrastructure, best practices, evidence communication, value, and systems approaches to improving health. These Collaboratives foster information sharing and cooperation across the health and health care system, explore emerging issues facing particular sectors of the health system, and harness the talent and expertise of the participants in practical efforts to advance the field.

WORKSHOP SCOPE AND OBJECTIVES

The workshop described in this publication was designed to initiate a comprehensive evaluation of the role of observational studies in contributing to the body of evidence for decision making in a learning health system (see Box 1-1). In setting the workshop's agenda, the planning committee intended individual participants to focus on

- Exploring the role of observational studies in the generation of evidence to guide clinical and health policy decisions in a learning health system with a focus on the care of the individual patient;
- Considering concepts of observational study design and analysis, emerging statistical methods, the opportunities and challenges of observational studies to supplement evidence from experimental methods, identify the heterogeneity of treatments, and provide estimates of effectiveness tailored to individual patients;
- Identifying stakeholder needs and the barriers hindering the broader application of evidence generated from observational studies to decision making;
- Engaging colleagues from disciplines typically underrepresented in discussions of clinical evidence; and
- Suggesting strategies for accelerating progress in the appropriate use of observational studies for the generation of evidence.

BOX 1-1
Statement of Task

An ad hoc committee will plan and guide the development of a 2-day public workshop to identify and explore issues, attitudes, and approaches to engaging expert stakeholders in exploring the role of observational studies in patient-centered and clinical effectiveness research. The purpose of the workshop is to initiate a comprehensive evaluation of the complementary roles of randomized controlled trials (RCTs) and observational studies and the use of patient-reported data, while looking ahead to the potential of very large sets of data from observational studies to transform the evidence generation needs of a continuously learning health care system. The committee will steer development of the agenda for the workshop, including the selection and invitation of speakers and discussants, and will moderate the discussions. The discussions will highlight fundamental questions defining real-world design; will discuss appropriate analytical approaches for a spectrum of studies, including those RCTs that closely resemble observational studies; and will consider policies, strategies, and procedures for data collection. The heterogeneity of patient responses to treatment will also be considered as it relates to the development of guidelines for individualized clinical care.

Through a series of expert presentations and discussions, workshop participants addressed how observational studies can be made to be more rigorous and internally valid, how to deal with bias, the use of observational studies to generalize the findings from RCTs to broader populations, and the prospects for the use of data from observational studies to evaluate treatment heterogeneity. In addition, presentations at the workshop considered whether observational studies have a role in predicting the response of individuals to treatment, which lies at the heart of personalized medicine. The final workshop session elicited perspectives from speakers with a variety of backgrounds and workshop participants on what the strategies going forward should be.

ORGANIZATION OF THE SUMMARY

This publication summarizes the discussions that occurred throughout the workshop, highlighting the key lessons presented, practical strategies, and the needs and opportunities for the use of observational studies in conjunction with RCTs in the context of a learning health care system. Chapter 2 discusses the role that observational studies can play in patient-centered outcomes research. Chapter 3 considers bias, Chapter 4 addresses key issues involved in the generalization of the results of RCTs to the broader population, and Chapter 5 highlights the role of observational studies in detecting the heterogeneous effects of treatment. Chapter 6 considers the prediction of individual treatment responses, and Chapter 7 discusses some of the common themes that emerged from the workshop discussions and strategies going forward.

REFERENCES

IOM (Institute of Medicine). 2009. *Transforming Clinical Research in the United States: Challenges and Opportunities: Workshop Summary.* Washington, DC: The National Academies Press.

IOM. 2012. *Best Care at Lower Cost: The Path to Continuously Learning Health Care in America.* Washington, DC: The National Academies Press.

Robert Wood Johnson Foundation. 2013. *Health Information Technology in the United States: Better Information Systems for Better Care.* Princeton, NJ: Robert Wood Johnson Foundation. http://www.rwjf.org/content/dam/farm/reports/reports/2013/rwjf406758 (accessed June 1, 2013).

2

Issues Overview for Observational Studies in Clinical Research

KEY SPEAKER THEMES

Goodman

- The choice between an observational study and a randomized controlled trial (RCT) is not binary.
- No algorithm exists for determining whether an observational study or an RCT is best for answering a specific question.
- The distinctions between observational studies and RCTs can be subtle, and interventions are changing in a way that requires studies with designs that can evaluate complex interventions.
- The design of a study needs to consider the context of a research program and the fact that different decision makers have different information needs.

To set the stage for the workshop's presentations and discussions, planning committee member Steven N. Goodman, Associate Dean for Clinical and Translational Research at the Stanford University School of Medicine, highlighted some of the issues involved in the use of clinical data, whether it be from a randomized controlled trial (RCT) or an observational study, to draw conclusions that are relevant to the health care decisions made by physicians and their patients.

PRESSING QUESTIONS FOR CONSIDERATION

With apologies to Charles Dickens, he portrayed the complexities of using data from the two types of clinical studies and the inability to resolve the intellectual differences that characterize the field of clinical trials today as being analogous to Paris in pre-Revolutionary France. "It was the best of times, it was the worst of times," Goodman began, "It was the age of Clinical Trials, it was the age of Observational Studies, it was the epoch of Data Mining, it was the epoch of Prespecification, it was the season of Discovery, it was the season of Decision, it was the spring of Effectiveness, it was the winter of Harms, we had Truth before us, we had Lies before us, we were all going direct to Causality, we were all going direct the other way—in short, the period was the present period, and some of its noisiest funders and policy makers insisted on its being perceived, for good or for evil, with a superlative degree of scientific rigor."

He then discussed a recent example from the popular press illustrating the challenges to the use of data from observational studies to develop treatment plans for individual patients. In this example, a statistician used one set of data to publish two papers whose findings on the health benefits of walking versus running appeared to contradict one another on the surface. However, the two papers were looking at different endpoints: one was looking at a surrogate endpoint, blood lipid levels, whereas the other was looking at weight loss. Goodman explained the resulting conundrum as such: the bottom-line advice for a specific patient depends on whether the patient wants to lose weight or control blood lipids, and that choice depends on multiple factors that were not included as variables in the study that generated the data.

Goodman cited the conflicting findings for hormone replacement therapy between a large number of observational studies and the RCT conducted by the Women's Health Initiative. Although as another example of why observational studies by themselves can provide misleading advice for patients, the former studies had demonstrated that hormone replacement therapy had a protective effect against heart attacks and the Women's Health Initiative study reported that hormone replacement therapy was associated a small increase in the risk for acute coronary outcomes. A reanalysis of the observational data pointed out important methodological flaws in the designs of both trials and found that the discrepancies could be resolved through a different conceptual framing of both the observational studies and RCTs (Hernán et al., 2008). According to Goodman, the insights from this reanalysis and the way in which it paired the two types of studies showed that "observational studies and RCTs are getting closer and closer. The choice between them is really not, in a sense, a choice between them but involves a lot of complicated trade-offs and questions about what each one reveals that the other one does not."

He then described what he called the foundational equation of epidemiology: Pr(outcome | $X = x$) = Pr[outcome | set($X = x$)]. He explained this equation to mean that the probability (Pr) of an outcome with an observed risk factor (X) is equal to the probability of that outcome when that risk factor is set equal to the same value (x). The equation can also be posed as a question: Is the observed effect the same as the effect seen when the variable is actively manipulated? If the answer to that question is "yes," then the result of the observational study can be transferred into the realm of practice.

Goodman noted that two prior reports—*Ethical and Scientific Issues in Studying the Safety of Approved Drugs* from the Institute of Medicine (IOM) (2012) and *Our Questions, Our Decisions: Standards for Patient-Centered Outcomes Research* from the Patient-Centered Outcomes Research Institute (PCORI) Methodology Committee (2012)—posed the same challenge facing the participants of the workshop described here, namely, determine the proper role for observational studies and RCTs in patient-centered outcomes research.

For the IOM study, two of the planning committee's charges were to (1) identify the strengths and weaknesses of the abilities of various approaches, including observational studies, patient registries, meta-analyses, meta-analyses of patient-level data, and RCTs, to generate evidence about safety questions and (2) determine what types of follow-up studies are appropriate, considering the speed, cost, and value of studies, to investigate different kinds of signals—detected before or after approval of a medication or device—and in what temporal order these studies should be conducted.

Goodman, who worked on both reports, noted that answering the second part of this charge was particularly difficult because experts can disagree for many legitimate reasons on the conclusions to be drawn from any particular dataset. As a result, no formulaic, algorithmic method is able to determine what types of studies are needed and in what temporal order studies should be conducted to answer a specific clinical question. Indeed, he explained, the decision to choose between an observational study and an RCT depends on multiple factors, including

- the size and nature of the signal,
- the size of the effect needed to justify a change in policy,
- temporal urgency,
- other potential causes of the outcome and whether the study will look for intended or unintended consequences,
- the quality and the availability of data,
- transportability, and
- the analytical approach as well as the study design.

In the report from PCORI, Goodman and his colleagues on the Institute's Methodology Committee came up with essentially the same recommendation presented in the IOM report: the choice between an observational study and an RCT is not binary, and no algorithm for determining which type of study is best for answering a specific question exists.

Rather than propose a specific translation table that would provide guidance to PCORI's board to determine research methods that are most likely to address each specific research question, the PCORI Methodology Committee developed a translation framework (see Figure 2-1) that considered the same factors identified in the IOM report. One key aspect of this framework is that it recommends that the research question and the trial design be kept separate to provide a focus for clarifying trade-offs. Another is that the framework recognize that many kinds of decision makers exist and that the information that the Centers for Medicare & Medicaid Services needs to make a decision about reimbursement issues is not going to be the same as the information that a clinician needs to make a decision at a patient's bedside. As a result, study design needs to consider the context of a research program and not the needs of one specific study. The framework also stresses that the study design must account for state-of-the-art research methodologies. Goodman cited his earlier example of the Women's Health

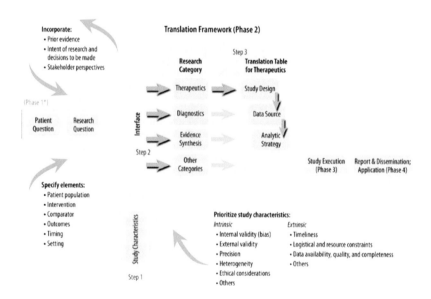

FIGURE 2-1 Phase 2 of PCORI translational framework to guide design of new clinical comparative effectiveness studies for specific research questions.
SOURCE: Reprinted with permission from PCORI.

Initiative study to support the importance of using the best methodologies available.

Goodman noted that in both of these reports the role and place of observational research in the world of therapeutics are central. His impression, based on his work on these two reports, is that there seems to be a strong need to apply the same, somewhat formulaic rules of evidence and design familiar to individuals in the world of evidence-based medicine to observational data. This need is apparent in the demand to create rules, or at least a social consensus, about what constitutes legitimate study designs for various questions. In his mind, the best approach is to articulate principles for discussion rather than frame the question of study design as a binary choice based on specific rules.

Turning to the perceived strengths and weakness of RCTs and observational studies, Goodman said that most positions on the strengths and weakness of RCTs and observational studies are extreme and tend to be caricatures of reality. He encouraged the workshop participants to not put themselves into doctrinaire camps along the lines that suggest that observational studies are generalizable and RCTs are not, that observational studies provide patient-centered individualized evidence and RCTs do not, that bias is minimal in RCTs but high in observational studies, or that data quality is high in RCTs but low in observational studies. For each one of these canards, he explained, study designs can make the two types of studies nearly equivalent. What is true, he said, is that the distinctions between observational studies and RCTs can be subtle and that interventions are changing in a way that requires that studies for the evaluation of these interventions have designs that are able to evaluate complex interventions. He noted that the field is facing a time when it has not only more data but also different types of data and more complex data. He added that the emphasis on transparency, reproducibility, and wider engagement in the scientific process is growing and that this emphasis can only benefit patient-centered outcomes research.

In his closing remarks, Goodman listed what he considered to be the central questions that he hoped the workshop would address:

- Does the method that is being talked about address the question we are really interested in?
- Does the method correctly estimate the effect for those to whom the results are applied? If not, how wrong is it?
- Does the method get the uncertainty right? If not, how wrong is it?
- Which of the approaches discussed at the workshop would be sound enough to guide a treatment decision? Would you bet a life on it? If not, could the field get there, and what would it take?

He also listed the key decisions that PCORI faces. First, it needs to determine what methodologies it should use in studies planned for today. Second, to determine the new methodologies in which it should invest, it needs to select the methodologies with the potential to yield the greatest benefits to patient-centered research. Finally, PCORI needs to establish the set of methods that will be taught to the next generation of those who will engage in patient-centered outcomes research.

DISCUSSION

During the discussion that followed Goodman's presentation, a number of participants stated the importance for researchers to first ask the right questions needed to make a clinically meaningful decision and then choose the study design and methodological tools to best answer those questions. Too often, participants commented, decision makers do not know the question that a study is answering and researchers do not delimit the question that they are asking or put a study into context, making the decision maker's job more difficult than it should be. Joel B. Greenhouse, professor of statistics at Carnegie Mellon University, wondered if it would be possible for the scientific community to reach a majority consensus as to what those important questions should be.

Harold Sox, professor of medicine at the Dartmouth Geisel School of Medicine, suggested that questions be framed in a way that generates data on uncertainties about outcomes. Such information would help patients and physicians make clinical decisions that have the right balance between potential harms and benefits for a particular patient. Mitchell H. Gail, senior investigator at the National Cancer Institute, responded by stating that the combination of RCTs and observational studies could provide an important understanding of how risks and benefits should be weighed across the baseline of people with various characteristics.

Several participants commented that the amount of data from observational studies that will be available to researchers will soon dwarf by several orders of magnitude the amount of data from RCTs. Marc L. Berger, vice president of real-world data and analytics at Pfizer, said that the real issue will not be whether observational data will be used but will be how they will be used. Sally C. Morton, professor and chair of the Department of Biostatistics in the Graduate School of Public Health at the University of Pittsburgh, added that many of the data that will be available will not come from designed studies and that different types of statistical methods will be needed to address what is essentially a model that is backward from the traditional situation in which data come from a study. James Robins, professor of epidemiology at Harvard University, proposed that the Internet data analytics community be evaluated to determine the questions to be answered when vast amounts of data have been collected but researchers do not have a question in mind. In particular, he mentioned that marginal structural modeling has the potential to be used to extrapolate patient-specific recommendations from large sets of clinical data.

Robert Temple, deputy director for clinical science at the Center for Drug Evaluation and Research, U.S. Food and Drug Administration, asked for examples of situations in which it was not possible to generalize the results of a clinical trial to a real population. In his experience, this has not, in fact, been the case. Goodman responded that the more context specific that a medical intervention is—and, in particular, when the intervention is something other than a drug-based therapy—the more likely it is that it will not be possible to generalize from the results of an RCT.

REFERENCES

Hernán, M. S., A. Alonso, R. Logan, F. Grodstein, K. B. Michels, W. C. Willett, J. E. Manson, and J. M. Robins. 2008. Observational studies analyzed like randomized experiments: An application to postmenopausal hormone therapy and coronary heart disease. *Epidemiology* 19(6):766–779.

IOM (Institute of Medicine). 2012. *Ethical and Scientific Issues in Studying the Safety of Approved Drugs*. Washington, DC: The National Academies Press.

Patient-Centered Outcomes Research Institute Methodology Committee. 2012. *Our Questions, Our Decisions: Standards for Patient-Centered Outcomes Research*. Draft Methodology Report. Washington, DC: Patient-Centered Outcomes Research Institute. http://pcori.org/assets/MethodologyReport-Comment.pdf (accessed May 14, 2013).

3

Engaging the Issue of Bias

KEY SPEAKER THEMES

Schneeweiss

- Accounting for bias is a major challenge confronting the use of observational data to gain important insights into real-world treatment effects.
- No single study design will satisfy all information needs of decision makers. A mix of studies could address the same question and complement each other in terms of internal and external validity, precision, timeliness, and cost in light of logistical constraints and ethics guidelines.

Small

- Instrumental variables can help correct for the effects of unmeasured confounders.
- Weak instrumental variables are useful for reliably detecting only large effects because of their sensitivity to even small biases.

Ryan

- Databases with health care data from observational studies contain valuable information, but the manner in which study results are generated and interpreted needs to be rethought to capitalize on the value of the databases.
- Study designs, including cohort, case-control, and self-controlled case series (SCCS), have varying performance characteristics when they are applied to different data sources or health outcomes of interest.

One of the major limits on the utility of observational studies is bias in various forms. Selection bias, for example, arises when a study population is not randomly selected from the target population, and measurement or information-related bias can result when data are missing from or misclassified in an electronic health record. To start the discussion on how to manage and control for bias in observational studies, Sebastian Schneeweiss, professor of medicine and epidemiology at Brigham and Women's Hospital and Harvard Medical School, provided an introduction to the issue of bias, laying the groundwork for presentations by Dylan Small, associate professor of statistics at the University of Pennsylvania, on instrumental variables, and Patrick Ryan, head of epidemiology analytics at Janssen Research and Development and participant in the Observational Medical Outcomes Partnership, on an empirical attempt to measure and calibrate for error in observational analyses. After comments by John B. Wong, professor of medicine at the Tufts University Sackler School of Graduate Biomedical Sciences, and Joel B. Greenhouse, professor of statistics at Carnegie Mellon University, an open discussion among the panelists and workshop attendees ensued.

AN INTRODUCTION TO THE ISSUE OF BIAS

In his short introduction to the subject of bias, Sebastian Schneeweiss described "effectiveness" to be a combination of the efficacy measured in randomized controlled trials and the suboptimal adherence and potential subgroup effects that reflect the reality of routine care. The appeal of observational studies lies in the potential to measure this reality through the linkage and analysis of electronic data that were generated in the process of providing care. The challenge with the use of such health care data, he explained, lies in accounting for the various forms of bias inherent in such data. These biases arise in large part because the investigator analyzing the data had no control over how and when the data were collected.

Surveillance-related biases occur when data collection is not uniform according to both how it was collected and the actual information collected. Missing information and misclassified information that are directly or indirectly related to the health outcomes of interest may cause bias. As an example of this type of bias, Schneeweiss described a study of new users and nonusers of statins that aimed to identify unintended clinical effects. At the baseline, the results of liver function tests were recorded for some 60 percent of new users, but those data were recorded for only 9 percent of nonusers.

Selection-related biases include confounding, in which patients with worse prognoses tend to be treated differently. Failure to fully adjust for those factors or proxies thereof leads to bias. Selection-related biases also arise when treatments change between the baseline and the time when the outcome is measured. The most common time-related bias, said Schneeweiss, is known as immortal time bias,[1] which occurs when the follow-up period is incorrectly attributed to groups exposed to a treatment or intervention, particularly in studies with nonuser groups.

Schneeweiss also discussed opportunities for managing some of these biases. Confounding, for example, can be managed by use of the naturally occurring variation in the nation's health care system. It should be possible, he said, to screen for naturally occurring variation through the use of propensity score analyses and apply instrumental variable analyses to use this variation for unbiased estimation, when appropriate (see the description of the presentation of Dylan Small on p. 20). Negative controls are useful as a diagnostic tool for residual confounding, if such controls can be established. As-treated versus intention-to-treat analyses can help describe a plausible range of bias by informative censoring, and inverse probability of discontinuous weighting can account for such bias, as can other methods that rely on characterizing the factors leading to a change in treatment.

Researchers have a growing appreciation, Schneeweiss said, for the idea of creating study portfolios that include multiple studies with different data sources, both primary and secondary, and different experimental designs. The issue here is to determine the optimal way to arrange multiple studies so that they complement each other according to their speed, validity, and generalizability and so that together they provide the most valid and comprehensive information for decision makers.

Regardless of which methods are used, no single study design will

---

[1] Immortal time refers to a span of time in the observation or follow-up period of a cohort during which the outcome under study could not have occurred. An incorrect consideration of this unexposed time period in the design or analysis will lead to immortal time bias. (S. Suissa. 2007. Immortal Time Bias in Pharmacoepidemiology. *American Journal of Epidemiology* 167(4):492–499.)

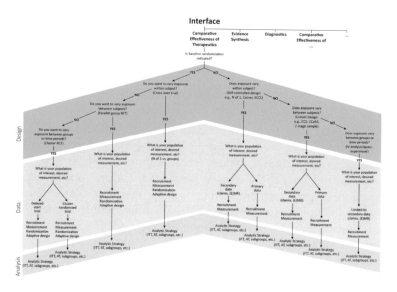

FIGURE 3-1 Study design decision tree for selecting design of studies of comparative effectiveness of therapeutics.
SOURCE: Reprinted with permission from PCORI.

satisfy the information needs of the decision maker. As a result, it is important to be transparent about the methods that are used to determine internal and external validity, precision, timeliness, and logistical constraints. Schneeweiss described the use of decision diagrams from the Patient-Centered Outcomes Research Institute (PCORI) Methodology Committee report (2012) (see Figure 3-1) that will encourage researchers to be more transparent about their implicit and explicit choices of study design, data, and analytical strategy, including their advantages and limitations. The use of flowcharts and decision diagrams might also help reduce the number of errors that result from investigators using data sources and methods incorrectly. Schneeweiss suggested that one opportunity for increasing transparency would be to develop an analytics infrastructure that allows other investigators to reanalyze data without having to move the data among investigators.

INSTRUMENTAL VARIABLES AND THEIR
SENSITIVITY TO UNOBSERVED BIASES

Dylan Small's presentation focused on the use of the instrumental variable method as one approach to controlling for unmeasured confounding. As an example, he discussed a 1994 study by Joshua Angrist and Alan Krueger of World War II veterans that examined the effect of military service on future earnings through the use of data measured in the 1980 census (Angrist and Krueger, 1994). At the time of that study, some studies suggested that military service would lower earnings because it interrupted an individual's education or career, but other research suggested that military service would raise earnings because the labor market might have favored veterans after World War II and the GI Bill might have increased veterans' education. The raw data on wages showed that World War II veterans earned about $4,500 more than nonveterans in 1980, suggesting that military service was associated with an increase in earnings. However, said Small, those data were not adjusted for any confounders. For example, someone who had been unhealthy or convicted of a crime would not have been eligible to serve in the military, and those factors, rather than military service per se, could account for lower later wages among nonveterans. "Health and criminal behavior are confounding variables, in that they are likely not comparable between the veterans and the nonveterans," said Small.

If all the confounders can be measured, Small continued, they can be adjusted for by regression or propensity scores, but most observational studies have unmeasured confounders. In fact, in the study of Angrist and Krueger (1994), neither health nor criminal behavior was measured in the census, and as a result, a regression of earnings on the basis of veteran status would produce a biased estimate.

The instrumental variables strategy is one approach to addressing unmeasured confounders. Again using the study of World War II veterans for purposes of illustration (Angrist and Krueger, 1994), Small explained that the idea is to identify a variable that is independent of the unobserved variables and does not have a direct effect on the outcome yet that will affect the treatment, which in this case is veteran status. "If we can find such a variable, then the idea is that we can extract the variation in the treatment from the instrument that is independent of the unmeasured confounders," said Small.

In a prototypical instrumental variable study, subjects are matched in pairs on the basis of whether or not the instrument encouraged an individual to get treatment. In this case, because birth is random, the matched pairs were individuals born in 1926 versus individuals born in 1928. Those born in 1926 were encouraged to become veterans by the year of their birth, while those born in 1928, who would have turned age 18 after the war had ended, were not encouraged to do so. Use of a two-stage squares method or permutation inference then produces the result that military service caused a substantial reduction of earnings of between $500 and $1,445 per year. As a check, this analysis was repeated with matched triples with men born in 1924, 1926, and 1928. This analysis matched men on the basis of the quarter of their birth, race, age, education up to 8 years, and location of birth; it also showed that military service decreased earnings.

One concern with this analysis, said Small, is that gradual long-term trends might play a hidden role in influencing wages. In the study of World War II veterans, gradual long-term trends in apprenticeship, education, employment, and nutrition might bias comparisons of workers born 2 years apart. A sensitivity analysis would ask how departures from random assignment of the instrumental variable of various magnitudes might alter the study's conclusions. In this case, sensitivity analysis showed that even a small amount of bias invalidates the inference that military service decreases earnings, but it does not invalidate the inference that military service raises earnings by $4,500 per year.

Small then discussed the strength of instrumental variables. A strong instrumental variable, he explained, has a strong effect on the treatment received. In the case of the earnings of World War II veterans, birth year is a strong variable if the years chosen are 1926 and 1928 because being born in 1926 substantially increases the chance that an individual would be a veteran compared with that for an individual born in 1928. Birth year is a weak variable if comparisons between 1924 and 1926 serve as the instrument because being born in 1924 raises only slightly the chance of being a veteran compared with that with being born in 1926. The effect obtained when a weak instrumental variable is chosen is increased variance. In this example, the 95 percent confidence interval for the effect of military service on income when a birth year of 1924 versus a birth year of 1926 is used as a comparator for 1928 was between a gain in income of $10,200 and a loss of income of $10,750, whereas the 95 percent confidence interval was an income between $500 and $1,445 lower for veterans.

Although it is possible to get a more precise inference with larger data sets, weaker instruments are still more sensitive to even small biases, Small explained. As a consequence, "weak instrumental variables can be dangerous to use and are probably only useful to detect enormous effects," he said. "Conversely, strong instrumental variables that might be moderately biased can be useful, as long as we do a sensitivity analysis to see if we have inferences that are robust enough to allowing for a moderate amount of bias." In closing, he listed some potential instrumental variables for health outcomes research (see Table 3-1), and he encouraged the community to work on creating useful instrumental variables.

TABLE 3-1 Strength of Potential Instrumental Variables in Health Outcomes Research

Potential Instrumental Variable	Strength
Differential distance to nearest provider of Treatment A vs. Treatment B	Weak or strong
Geographic or hospital preference for Treatment A vs. Treatment B	Weak or strong
Physician preference for Treatment A vs. Treatment B	Weak or strong
Calendar time (one treatment may become more common over time)	Weak or strong
Genetic variants	Usually weak
Timing of admission to hospital	Weak or strong
Insurance plan coverage for Treatment A vs. Treatment B	Weak or strong
Randomized encouragement at point of care for Treatment A vs. Treatment B when no clear-cut choice exists	Potentially strong

SOURCE: Reprinted with permission from Dylan Small.

AN EMPIRICAL APPROACH TO MEASURING AND CALIBRATING FOR ERROR IN OBSERVATIONAL ANALYSES

Before starting his formal presentation, Patrick Ryan noted that he was giving this talk on behalf of the Observational Medical Outcomes Partnership (OMOP) and that all of the data he would be discussing are available publicly at the Partnership's website (http://omop.org). He then described what he called a framework for thinking about how to measure bias and how to quantify how well observational studies perform. The intent of this framework, he explained, is to use the information that it produces as the context for interpreting observational studies and to adjust and calibrate analytical estimates to be more in line with expectations.

As an example, Ryan discussed a study described in a paper published in the *British Journal of Clinical Pharmacology* that examined the risk of gastrointestinal bleeding in association with the drug clopidogrel (Opatrny et al., 2008). That paper described the results of a nested case-control observational study conducted using the United Kingdom's General Practice Research Database. Ryan characterized the study as a typical observational study. In this particular case, the authors found that clopidogrel increased the risk of gastrointestinal bleeding with an adjusted rate ratio of 2.07 and a 95 percent confidence interval that spanned from 1.66 to 2.58. "How much can we believe that there is a doubling of risk?" asked Ryan. Framed another way, he wondered how far away the adjusted rate ratio of 2.07 is from the true value as a result of bias. For clarification, he defined the term "coverage" to be the probability that the confidence interval contains the true effect, which, for 95 percent confidence intervals, would be the effect expected 95 percent of the time.

One way to qualitatively assess the performance of a method would be to use three to four negative controls pairs (drug and outcome pairs that have been shown not to have an association) in addition to the target outcome pair, as a means of assessing the plausibility of the result from an observational analysis. If the same outcome was not found for those negative controls, "maybe in some qualitative way, you would feel better about the plausibility of your effect," said Ryan. What OMOP has been doing instead is use a large sample of negative and positive controls to empirically measure analysis operating characteristics and use those to calibrate study findings. For this example, OMOP implemented a nested case-control study with a standardized approach to matching cases and controls with a standard set of inclusion and exclusion criteria. As a data source, OMOP used a large U.S. administrative claims database, and the analysis estimated that clopidogrel increased the risk of gastrointestinal bleeding with an adjusted odds ratio of 1.86 and a 95 percent confidence interval of 1.79 to 1.93. Ryan said the tighter confidence interval was in large part a result of the larger data sample size that OMOP used in the analysis.

The OMOP team next took the same standardized implementation of that method and consistently applied it across a network of databases to a large sample of negative and positive controls. For gastrointestinal bleeding, the OMOP team specifically identified 24 drugs that it believed were associated with bleeding and 67 drugs for which they could find no evidence to suggest that the drug might be related to gastrointestinal bleeding, on the basis of product labeling and information in the literature. For these negative controls, if the 95 percent confidence interval was properly calibrated, then 95 percent, or 62 of 65, of the relative risk estimates would cover a relative risk of 1. In fact, the analysis found that only 29 of the 65 negative controls covered a relative risk of 1 and the error distribution demonstrated a positive bias and substantial variability for this case-control method, the same used in the clopidogrel study (see Figure 3-2).

A variety of measures can be used to measure the accuracy of a method, explained Ryan, but one of the challenges with the measurement of accuracy is that it is possible to make assumptions about benchmarking of an estimate only relative to the truth. For negative controls, the assumption is that they have a relative risk of 1, but it is not possible to assume the estimate of the effect for positive controls. Another approach is to measure discrimination, which is the probability that an estimate from an observational study can distinguish between no effect and a positive effect regardless of the size of the effect. Sensitivity and specificity are additional measures of accuracy, in which sensitivity is the percentage of positive controls that meet

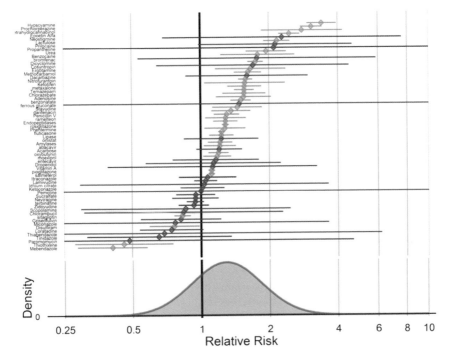

FIGURE 3-2 Case-control estimates for gastrointestinal bleeding negative controls. The y-axis lists the 65 negative controls, and the x-axis denotes relative risk. Values in orange are statistically significant; values in blue are not. The error distribution (bottom) demonstrates a positive bias of this method and substantial variability. SOURCE: Reprinted with permission from Patrick Ryan.

a decision threshold of dichotomous criteria, and specificity is the percentage of negative controls that do not meet this same decision threshold.

When Ryan and his colleagues compared the accuracy of cohort and self-controlled designs using different methods, databases, and outcomes, they found that each type of analysis has its own error distribution and all methods have low coverage probability. He said that from here one can take one of two directions: either improve the methods to reduce the magnitude of error or quantify the error and use it to adjust the estimates of the effect through empirical calibration. Instead of having a theoretical null distribution based only on sampling variability, it should be possible to use the empirical null distribution based on the uncertainty measured from negative controls when the method is applied to the data source. Application of this approach to the clopidogrel and gastrointestinal bleeding example produces a new range for the adjusted odds ratio of 0.79 to 4.57, which Ryan explained means that the results are not statistically significant and that it is not possible to rule out the possibility that the effect is not larger than 4. Calibration, he said, does not influence discrimination, but it does tend to improve bias, mean squared error, and coverage.

Concluding his talk, Ryan said that observational studies contain valuable information but that there is a need to rethink how study results are interpreted to capitalize on the value of the databases. One approach, which OMOP is taking, is to conduct a systematic exploration of negative and positive controls, both to measure the operating characteristics of a given method and to use that measurement to revise initial estimates and consider the true uncertainty observed in those studies.

COMMENT

John B. Wong noted that the use of empirical adjustment in the methods that OMOP is developing has a real potential to reduce false-positive and false-negative results. He also remarked on the importance of Small's work with instrumental variables and their use in quantifying the degree of bias associated with unmeasured confounding. He added that this work demonstrated that two-stage least-squares analysis should not be used with weak instrumental variables, that an increased sample size can produce useful results if the instrumental variable is valid, and that it is important to explicitly examine the sensitivity of a weak instrumental variable to biases.

Joel B. Greenhouse then reminded the workshop participants that this is not the first time that researchers have discussed how to best use observational studies. In particular, he mentioned the work of Jerome Cornfield, performed in the 1950s, that demonstrated a causal association between smoking and lung cancer (Cornfield, 2012). He recommended two papers originally published in 1959 and recently reprinted in *Statistics in Medicine* and the *International Journal of Epidemiology* (Cornfield, 2012; Cornfield et al., 2009). The first paper, said Greenhouse, outlined a defense of the evidence generated from observational studies and addressed every issue being discussed at the workshop (Cornfield, 2012). The second paper, which informed the Surgeon General's report on smoking, looked at every alternative explanation for a link between smoking and lung cancer and found that none sufficed (Cornfield et al., 2009).

Greenhouse then noted the value of the methods that Ryan and his colleagues at OMOP are developing. Given Small's presentation, he questioned the value of the instrumental variable approach for patient-centered outcomes research, particularly when a decision maker is trying to answer the question of what therapy is appropriate for a specific patient. He concluded his comments by noting that the strategy of conducting observational studies has not changed from Cornfield's time. It is critical to start with thoughtful objectives, including the identification of the target population of interest, and a well-designed study that uses appropriate measurements and information from multiple data sources to investigate and eliminate alternative hypotheses.

DISCUSSION

Session moderator, Michael S. Lauer, director of the Division of Prevention and Population Sciences at the National Heart, Lung, and Blood Institute, asked the panel if it was ever acceptable today to do a straightforward regression analysis of observational data. Schneeweiss answered that everyone attending the workshop should agree that one analysis of any kind by itself is no longer sufficient. He said that the biggest challenge today, which was highlighted by Small's and Ryan's presentations, is to ensure that investigators are properly using these new methods. Wong agreed with that assessment and noted that two papers on how to conduct and report on studies through the use of instrumental variables would be appearing in the May 2013 issue of the journal *Epidemiology*. Greenhouse added that, in addition to multiple methods, multiple studies conducted in different contexts and with different populations are needed. Small commented that he would like to see some thought put into how to report sensitivity analyses in a way that would be useful to clinicians and decision makers.

Nancy Santanello, vice president for epidemiology at Merck, asked the panel if any of the methods that they discussed or know about deals specifically with misclassification bias or provides a measure of the reliability of the data in large databases. Ryan said that the work that he discussed does not deal with misclassification separately but, rather, bundles all of the unmeasured confounders into one composite measure of error that is integrated into the subsequent analysis.

Steven N. Goodman asked the panelists to discuss what they thought the most effective investments would be for further development of these methodologies. Ryan said that investment in methods development is needed and that PCORI should invest in new approaches to the use of instrumental variables and large-dimensional regressions, as well as in methods to evaluate the methods that are being developed. As an example, he said that he would like to see instrumental variable methods implemented, along with an assessment of how they work in practice. Schneeweiss agreed that the field is now at a place where it understands how these methods work and that their performance should be assessed; however, Schneeweiss thought that the bigger issue is that even the best methods used incorrectly will yield bad results. He suggested that it would be useful to simulate and insert into a data source a known association and to then try to identify that association as a "gold standard" for performance, an idea that Wong seconded.

Small said that he thought that it would be useful to validate performance in specific settings of some common types of instrumental variables, such as physician prescribing preferences or geographic variations. He thought that such studies could provide information on the types of data that need to be measured and collected to make these instruments valid in other settings. Dean Follmann, branch chief and associate director for biostatistics at the National Institutes of Health, thought that with many of the new databases being developed an opportunity exists to also consider new types of study designs that build context-specific instrumental variables into the studies. As an example, he proposed a hypothetical trial of a human immunodeficiency virus vaccine in Malawi in which the country's 12 provinces would be randomized and then the vaccine would be administered to individuals in the randomized provinces at different times of the year. This would essentially create a trial with a built-in instrumental variable.

Changing the subject, Sheldon Greenfield, executive codirector of the Health Policy Research Institute at the University of California, Irvine, asked for workshop attendees to comment on the idea that observational studies should be held to some standard in terms of the variables included in those studies. In particular, when confounders are known but not available in a dataset, should investigators be required to find those variables or proxies for those variables in other data sets or even the original dataset? Greenhouse voiced the opinion that PCORI should invest in ensuring that databases with data from observational studies have the variables that are needed to do the types of investigations that will help clinicians and decision makers. Wong noted that the retrospective collection of data on unmeasured confounders is somewhat difficult and that doing so introduces new biases into any analysis.

A workshop participant from a remote site asked the panel to comment on the effect on bias of the requirement that PCORI must involve patients and other stakeholders in the design of research, given the lack of technical knowledge among patients. Lauer noted that innumeracy is a problem not just among patients but also among many clinicians. Wong said that he believes that patients can play an important role in deciding what outcomes are important so that investigators can then use the methods presented here, for example, to design their studies to address those outcomes.

Mark A. Hlatky, professor and Stanford Health Policy Fellow in the Department of Health Research and Policy at Stanford University, asked the panelists to provide some guidance on when to decide that a particular method is not yielding useful information. Ryan said that his approach is to use multiple methods to determine which method has the most desirable operating characteristics, discriminates best, has less bias, and has the best coverage. All things being equal, Ryan said that he would pick the analytical method that has the preferred operating characteristics. Small said that for the instrumental variable method, it would be useful to do more power sensitivity analyses for observational studies that identify how much statistical power is needed to detect an effect yet still be insensitive to a bias of some plausible magnitude. If no power to detect an effect that allows even a small amount of bias exists, then it would useful to find some other study design or database for that study.

Santanello asked Ryan if the methods that OMOP developed to look at safety could be applied to look at comparative effectiveness. Ryan replied that the same data sources are used to examine safety and comparative effectiveness, so the same types of analytical strategies should work. The issue, he continued, is to decide how to create the reference set of positive and negative controls in the context of comparative effectiveness rather than safety.

REFERENCES

Angrist, J., and A. B. Krueger. 1994. Why do World War II Veterans earn more than nonveterans? *Journal of Labor Economics* 85(5):1065–1087.

Cornfield, J. 2012. Principles of research: 1959. *Statistics in Medicine* 31(24):2760–2768.

Cornfield, J., W. Haenszel, E. C. Hammond, A. M. Lilienfeld, M. B. Shimkin, and E. L. Wynder. 2009. Smoking and lung cancer: Recent evidence and a discussion of some questions. *International Journal of Epidemiology* 38(5):1175–1191.

Opatrny, L., J. A. Delaney, and S. Suissa. 2008. Gastro-intestinal haemorrhage risks of selective serotonin receptor antagonist therapy: A new look. *British Journal of Clinical Pharmacology* 66(1):76–81.

4

Generalizing Randomized Clinical Trial Results to Broader Populations

---

KEY SPEAKER THEMES

Califf

- Observational studies can be powerful tools for generalizing the results of randomized controlled trials (RCTs), but only if they are well designed to answer specific clinical questions.
- To maximize the ability of observational studies to generalize the results of RCTs, create a three-dimensional informatics infrastructure comprising electronic health records; high-quality, granular, and detailed registries; and patient-reported outcomes.

Hernán

- Ask the right questions so that comparisons of RCTs and observational studies are done with the right analytical tools.
- The terms "effectiveness" and "efficacy" are too vague to define the questions of interest.
- For comparative effectiveness research, RCTs will need to be analyzed as though they were the results of observational studies.

Kaizar

- When a synthesis across different types of data is being conducted, it is important to examine all of the available evidence to ensure that any inferences are consistent, explainable, and applicable to the identified population of interest.
- Observational studies can be used to generalize from RCTs, but such a generalization should rely on an analytical framework that explicitly describes the parameters estimable from each type of data and the relationships among these parameters.

Randomized controlled trials (RCTs) use a rigorous experimental design to evaluate the average overall benefit and risk of a specific therapy when it is used by a narrowly defined, select group of patients treated under carefully controlled conditions. Because most RCT protocols limit enrollment eligibility to select groups of individuals, application of the findings from an RCT to broader populations can be problematic, particularly if the treatment effect differs for those who are not represented by the population chosen for an RCT.

Robert M. Califf, vice chancellor for clinical research at the Duke University Medical Center, started the session by reviewing the challenges that the medical community faces in translating the results of RCTs to broader populations. Miguel A. Hernán, professor of epidemiology at Harvard University, showed how the utility of both RCTs and observational studies can be increased when the right clinical questions are asked before the studies are designed, and Eloise E. Kaizar, associate professor in the Department of Statistics at The Ohio State University, considered whether it is possible to generalize the findings of studies designed to evaluate efficacy to inform effectiveness. William S. Weintraub, the John H. Ammon Chair of Cardiology at Christiana Care Health Services, and Constantine Frangakis, professor in the Department of Biostatistics at the Johns Hopkins Bloomberg School of Public Health, commented on the three presentations and joined the panel for an open discussion with the workshop attendees.

INTRODUCTION TO THE ISSUE

To start the session, Robert M. Califf provided a framework for thinking about the issue of efficacy and effectiveness in a broader population. The first question that must be asked is, Does the therapy work at all, and can it be distinguished from placebo or the standard of care? The best way to answer this question is to conduct an RCT. Once efficacy is established, clinical studies are needed to determine how the treatment should be used, the types of patients who should use it, and how long it should be used. The traditional approach to those issues involved subgroup analysis, an approach that Califf says is flawed because of the small amount of data for most subgroups in most clinical trials.

Califf commented on the way in which the standard of practice in acute cardiac care came to be in the United States, noting that all the foundational studies were conducted by entering patients into clinical trials as soon as they entered the hospital emergency room. This approach led to tens of thousands of people being randomized into clinical trials, and it generated findings that were clear-cut, making it easy to develop clinical practice guidelines.

What has become clear is that these guidelines are effective only when they are followed. To prove this fact, Califf discussed large national studies showing that for every 10 percent improvement in adherence to what worked in RCTs, mortality decreased by 11 percent. Similar results have been seen in heart failure patients, in which each 10 percent improvement in adherence to composite care recommended by clinical guidelines reduced mortality by 13 percent.

In contrast, erythropoietin prescribing guidelines for kidney dialysis patients were determined from dozens of what Califf called "shoddy" observational studies. These studies purported to show that high-dose erythropoietin benefited patients with chronic kidney disease who were on dialysis, and the medical community went along with those recommendations. When Califf and others conducted RCTs of erythropoietin, the results were distressing: patients on high-dose erythropoietin experienced higher mortality and worse clinical outcomes than patients receiving low doses of the drug. The medical community, said Califf, had been misled by "dozens of mutually reinforcing observational studies."

In his opinion, the situation with erythropoietin is likely to become more common in everyday clinical practice unless the health care community takes a wholly systematic approach to evaluation of the results of different types of trials that are used to demonstrate efficacy and effectiveness. The challenge is to move from a situation in which validity and generalizability are low to one in which both are high.

He then discussed another example of a trial in which the average result was not broadly applicable. In this case, a worldwide trial compared the efficacy of the well-established anticlotting agent clopidogrel with that of a new drug, ticagrelor (Wallentin et al., 2009). The primary endpoint of this study was the time to cardiovascular death, myocardial infarction, or stroke. The results showed that ticagrelor lowered the cumulative incidence of major cardiac events and reduced total mortality, both in the worldwide population and in every predefined subgroup except one: patients in North America. A sophisticated statistical analysis based on observational analysis suggested that the reason for this difference was that North Americans take more aspirin than everyone else.

In his closing comments, Califf said the answer to the problem of how to generalize from RCTs lies in creation of a fundamental informatics infrastructure that forms a three-dimensional matrix. Along one dimension are the data from every American's electronic health record, whereas the second dimension consists of high-quality, granular, and detailed registries created by every relevant patient advocacy group and professional society. The third dimension is patient-reported outcomes recorded and reported by use of the ubiquitous cell phone.

GENERALIZING THE RIGHT QUESTION

Miguel A. Hernán began his presentation by stating that while observational studies address important challenges in comparative effectiveness research, observational studies do have some strengths. "They are faster, less expensive, [and] have fewer ethical problems, and the results may be more transportable to other populations," said Hernán. Observational studies are more transportable, he explained, because the patients in such studies are more similar to real-life patients and they are often followed for longer periods of time. In addition, the treatments being compared are implemented under more realistic settings in an observational study. What would happen, Hernán asked, "if randomized trials and observational studies had the same patients, the same follow-up, and the same type of interventions? Would they be answering the same question?" He would argue that the answer is "no" because the two types of studies are not typically analyzed in the same way.

"We usually consider a randomized trial and an observational follow-up study as two different types of follow-up designs, but they may actually be very similar, except that the randomized trial treatment is randomized at baseline," said Hernán. "We can think of randomized clinical trials as follow-up studies with baseline randomization." If that is the case, he argued, it might be more useful to classify studies according to whether they had baseline randomization, without automatic assignment of greater validity to follow-up studies with baseline randomization. For example, in large simple trials and so-called pragmatic trials, the benefits of baseline randomization can be overshadowed by high rates of noncompliance and loss of patients to follow-up, and typically, data are not collected to adjust for these biases.

Regardless, the analysis of results from studies with these two types of designs differs, he explained. Most randomized trials use intent-to-treat analysis (ITT), whereas most observational studies use as-treated analysis, to enable adjustment of baseline confounding. Both study designs, however, require adjustment for postbaseline confounding and for selection bias that may result from patients lost to follow-up after the baseline, neither of which is controlled by randomization.

The purpose of the ITT design is to identify the effect of being assigned to a treatment independently of what happens after the baseline. The goal is to compare those who are assigned to Treatment A and continue with follow-up until the end of the study with those who are assigned to Treatment B and continue with follow-up until the end of the study. The analysis may require adjustment for selection bias because of differential loss to follow-up, and that adjustment requires information on postbaseline confounders.

Hernán added that follow-up studies with baseline randomization may also want to examine the effect of the treatment as specified in the study protocol. In this case, the goal is to determine the effect of Treatment A over the entire course of the study, unless the patient experiences toxic effects, versus Treatment B over the entire course of the study, unless the patient experiences toxic effects. A follow-up study with baseline randomization can also aim to quantify the effect of some treatment or some form of that treatment and the effect of that treatment received in some other way that is not specified in the protocol. Again, what happens after the baseline is not controlled by randomization in either of these study designs and an adjustment for time-varying confounding and selection bias will need to be made. However, in most reported studies, said Hernán, investigators do not adjust for time-varying, postbaseline variables.

Turning to the subject of efficacy and effectiveness, Hernán said that these terms are probably useful in simple settings with short-term interventions, but they become ambiguous in complex settings with sustained interventions over long periods. Rather, he said, what would be more informative is an explicit definition of the interventions that define the causal effect of interest. He noted that an ITT effect does not necessarily measure effectiveness in the real world, whereas a per protocol effect may measure effectiveness but not, in general, efficacy. What would be useful, he said, would be to define the observational analogs of ITT and per protocol effects. Having such definitions would provide an idea of what questions can be generalized. A good start toward such definitions, he said, are the new user designs that aim to estimate ITT effects in observational studies.

Hernán briefly reviewed the methods that he and his colleagues used to reanalyze the data on the effects of hormone therapy on the risk of heart disease (Hernán et al., 2008). Most observational studies conducted in the 1980s and 1990s had found that women currently on hormone replacement therapy had a 30 percent lower risk of developing heart disease than did women who were not on hormone replacement therapy (Stampfer and Colditz, 1991). Then, the Women's Health Initiative RCT found that women initiating hormone replacement therapy had a 20 percent increased risk of developing heart disease compared with the risk for those who were given placebo (Manson et al., 2003). Hernán explained that these studies were asking two very different questions and that the results were not comparable. The question asked by the randomized trial was, what is the heart disease risk in women assigned to initiation of hormone therapy compared with women assigned to no initiation of hormone therapy? The observational study asked, what is the heart disease risk in women who are currently taking hormone therapy compared with women who are not? When he and his colleagues reanalyzed the observational data to estimate the analog of the ITT effect measured in the RCT, they found that risk was elevated in the first 2 years of therapy but that there was no elevated risk in women who were within 10 years of menopause.

Although this reanalysis did not produce exactly the same result, the discrepancy was far smaller because both analyses were asking the same ITT question, which compares groups based on their baseline randomization. However, one problem with the ITT study was that close to 40 percent of the women did not comply with the protocol. When these data were reanalyzed to identify the per protocol effect, which is based on whether participants fulfilled the protocol, the results from the RCT and observational studies were also similar.

Hernán then discussed an example of analysis of the findings of an RCT as if it was an observational study (Hernán et al., 2008). In this case, the data came from the Women's Health Initiative RCT, and the reanalysis attempted to estimate a per protocol effect by using inverse probability weighting and by taking advantage of the data that were collected after randomization. When the data were analyzed in the manner described, the per protocol hazard ratio was 1.7 for breast cancer. whereas the intent-to-treat hazard ratio was 1.2. Hernán characterized the difference as large and significant for a woman who is considering whether to go on hormone replacement therapy. As Hernán put it, the relevant question for a woman planning to take therapy is, what is the effect of hormone replacement therapy on women who actually complied with the therapy and not what is the effect of hormone replacement therapy on women who enrolled in a clinical trial?

In conclusion, Hernán said that the question of interest must be stated clearly for both RCTs and observational studies as far as whether the goal is to get an ITT effect, a per protocol effect, or other effects. Once the question is in hand, then the analysis of both RCTs and observational studies should be the same, except for adjustment for baseline confounding. He also reiterated his earlier comment that the terms "effectiveness" and "efficacy" are too vague to define the questions of interest.

USE OF OBSERVATIONAL STUDIES TO
DETERMINE GENERALIZABILITY OF RCTs

After agreeing with Hernán that efficacy and effectiveness are indeed vague concepts in terms of formulating research questions, Eloise E. Kaizar said that these terms are useful for classifying the types of effects that investigators should think about when designing their analyses. In the development setting, the term "efficacy" helps define the best population of individuals to be treated to design the most cost-efficient trial, to have the greatest chance of showing a positive treatment effect, if one exists, and to avoid recruiting people who might be harmed by the treatment. In the policy-setting arena, thinking about effectiveness brings a focus on the population or subpopulation that needs to be studied.

She then turned to the question at hand: is it possible to generalize information from studies designed to evaluate efficacy to inform effectiveness? She first defined two populations: the target population and the trial population. A target population is the population of all individuals for whom a treatment may be considered for its intended purpose, whereas a trial population is a theoretical population that consists of all individuals who would be eligible to enroll in an RCT. Although it is clear that it is straightforward to generalize about the trial population from the RCT analysis, the key is to define or model how the trial population relates to the target population.

These two populations can be considered in relation to each other in a number ways, she continued. In the best-case scenario, the trial population is a simple random sample from the target population. If this is the case, the distribution of baseline variables would be identical between the two populations and the distribution of outcome variables would be logically related. Comparison of the distribution of baseline variables in trial participants and a representative sample of the target population from administrative or survey sources could identify discrepancies or evidence against the use of a simple random sample from the target population. For example, in a study of suicidality associated with antidepressant use, the RCTs suggested that taking antidepressants was associated with a risk of increased rates of suicidality among adolescents (Greenhouse et al., 2008). She and her colleagues thought it reasonable to assume that more subjects enrolled in the trials would be taking antidepressants than in the population at large, so they should observe a higher rate of suicidality in the trials than in the observational data. That was not the case, however, providing evidence that in this case they could not treat the trial population as a simple random sample from the target population.

The next and more complicated way to relate the two populations is to think of the trial population as a weighted sample of the target population. The idea is that the trial population has a representative sample but that the distribution of attributes is different than in the target population. Reweighting schemes include probability sampling methods from the survey sampling research community, such as poststratification or propensity-based standardization. However, patients are not recruited into trials as a weighted sample, given the number of inclusion and exclusion criteria imposed on the trial population, and studies have consistently shown, Kaizar noted, that it is usual for RCTs to include at most half of the target population as a result of eligibility criteria. What is not known, though, is whether these exclusions are important for generalization from the results of RCTs.

The bottom line, she said, is that once an analysis moves to a population outside of the trial population, it becomes an extrapolation, which then requires additional steps to determine if extrapolation is reasonable. For example, sensitivity analysis can estimate what the effect size needs to be in the excluded subpopulation for the inference from the trial population to change for the target population. If that effect size is large, then the extrapolation is likely to be reasonable. Another approach, which was discussed by earlier speakers, is to compare data from an RCT to data from parallel observational studies. One way to do such a comparison, said Kaizar, is to apply the exclusion criteria to data representative of the target population through the use of methods based on a cross-design synthesis framework, which combines results from studies with complementary designs (U.S. General Accounting Office, 1992). The idea here, she explained, is to stratify the target population by those represented in the trial and those not represented in the trial. This approach assumes that no residual confounding exists within subpopulations or that residual confounding is separate from the exclusion criteria. She recommended that this type of approach be incorporated into Phase IV explorations to promote a learning health care environment.

As an example, she briefly discussed an RCT of insulin pump use and the generalization of findings to the target population (Doyle et al., 2004). The RCT showed, as expected, that in the very controlled environment of the trial, insulin pump use was more effective than self-administration of insulin at improving metabolic control, as measured by blood hemoglobin A1c levels. However, the criteria for this trial excluded the very population that would most likely benefit from automated insulin administration: those patients who do not check their blood glucose levels regularly. In this case, the RCT likely underestimated the average effect size in the target population, which Kaizar noted was probably of interest to insurance companies that may be more willing to pay for these pumps.

In concluding her presentation, Kaizar said the point that she wanted to emphasize was that when one is synthesizing across types of data, it is important to examine all of the available evidence to ensure that any inferences are consistent or explainable. She said, too, that the field needs to start thinking about how to work with multiple treatments. Stratification, she said in closing, "is very much an artifact of believing that the people who are in the trial represent everyone in that population who would be eligible. This is a bit naïve, in that patients also opt out of the trial for various reasons that we certainly cannot define a priori." She noted that it is important to start thinking about how to capture that phenomenon, perhaps thinking about population membership as a more fuzzy or soft classification.

COMMENT

In his comments, William S. Weintraub said that he heard two important messages. The first, from Hernán, is to ask the right questions so that comparisons between RCTs and observational studies are done with the right analytical tools and are in fact comparing apples to apples. The second, from Kaizar, is that observational studies can be used to generalize from RCTs, but only if the confounders are the same, and if they are not, then an analytical framework must be used to account for any differences. As an example of the latter, he cited RCTs that showed that revascularization was beneficial for relatively young patients with acute coronary syndrome. The issue was whether this effect was generalizable to older populations. In this case, the confounders were not the same: elderly patients in the RCTs were less sick than those in the target population.

Weintraub also discussed an example in which the results from RCTs and observational studies did not match. In this case, a large observational study of hundreds of thousands of subjects undergoing revascularization showed a survival advantage for those who received drug-eluting stents compared with the survival for those who received bare metal stents, but no difference in repeat revascularization. In contrast, the RCTs showed the opposite: a benefit in terms of revascularization but not in terms of mortality. In this case, he said, size did not overcome what were in fact large and unaccounted for biases in the observational studies. As a result, the findings of the RCT were the more believable of the two types of studies.

To illustrate the power of use of a combination of study results to make more generalizable conclusions, he described a study funded by the U.S. Food and Drug Administration (FDA) to examine the comparative safety of different stents (Weintraub et al., 2012). The original RCTs were small and were designed to demonstrate efficacy, so Weintraub and his colleagues combined the data from the RCTs with data from a prospective observational study and a large patient registry. Using data from some 60,000 patients, they found that one of the devices had an odds ratio for vascular complications of 4, which was high enough to be believable and exclude the possibility of treatment selection bias. "That device was off of the market within a couple of weeks," said Weintraub. "To me, that was one of the triumphs of comparative effectiveness research."

As a final comment, Weintraub noted that the use of patient registries is good for comparing quality of care and treatment adherence but that too often they are used to compare outcomes. Their use for comparison of outcomes presents a danger, however, because of the confounders resulting from the variations in the evaluation of thousands of health care providers. He made a plea to create registries that are coupled with electronic health records (EHRs) to address this issue.

Constantine Frangakis said that an important point that Hernán made was that investigators need to pay close attention to the possible differences that a randomized study and an observational study may have in their standard way of dealing with estimates, particularly given that most RCTs use an ITT protocol and most observational studies analyze data on an as-treated basis. Another potential issue, said Frangakis, is that in an RCT, it is often possible to ask participating physicians about deviations from the therapeutic protocol, something that cannot be done with observational studies. Therefore, the model being used in the two studies would be different in ways that are not identifiable. He added that post-treatment confounders make it difficult to use observational studies to generalize from RCTs. Regarding Kaizar's talk, Frangakis said that he thought covariates, propensity scores, and extrapolation are useful and important analytical considerations.

DISCUSSION

Session moderator Harold C. Sox asked Kaizar if he understood her correctly that extraction of excluded patients from the target population and comparison of the remaining subjects with those in the RCT provide a more valid estimate of the treatment effect in the target population minus those who were excluded from participating in the RCT. She replied that his understanding was correct. She added that it is necessary to adjust for the population with data from the observational study to average the effects in the two subpopulations and argued that the result would be a reasonable effect size in the target population. She reiterated that such extrapolation always involves the making of assumptions that must be tested for validity.

Sox then asked the panel if it is now standard practice for randomized trials to have an observational cohort representing patients who were excluded. Weintraub answered that the answer was "no." If anything, he indicated, because of financial constraints, this is being done less frequently now than it was 30 years ago. Robert M. Califf added that the only group that he knows of that does this routinely is the Society of Thoracic Surgeons, largely because it maintains a registry database of nearly everyone who undergoes a cardiothoracic procedure in North America. This registry enables investigators conducting RCTs to know who was randomized to the trial population and who was not. He also noted that the Health Systems Research Collaboratory of the National Institutes of Health is now conducting seven clinical trials using EHRs in a similar manner.

Califf commented that he believes that the field is in transition right now and that as a researcher who conducts clinical trials, he would be dubious about the result of any observational study with an odds ratio of less than 2 to 3. However, the situation will improve greatly when the field moves into the era in which everyone has an EHR. "In my view, we just got to live through this really agonizing period of time," he said. He also added that he believes that large, expensive, data-intensive RCTs are going to be a thing of the past when this transition is complete.

Sean Hennessy, associate professor of epidemiology at the University of Pennsylvania, asked Hernán whether the instrumental variable approach would be the best for comparison of data from an RCT with as-treated observational data. For simple studies, Hernán said, instrumental variables work well, but they are not developed enough for use with more complex studies that have time-varying confounding and selection bias, for example.

Joe V. Selby asked Kaizar if it would be reasonable, when one is planning an observational study designed to extend findings from an RCT, to build into the cohort of the observational study the same group that was in the RCT. Kaizar agreed that that was a good idea, particularly for the first observational study of a particular problem, but that the study should also be designed to collect data from a wide range of patients.

Califf remarked that one problem that frustrates him is the lack of information on observational studies that have been conducted but that failed to produce the desired result and so were never published. He hopes that the Patient-Centered Outcomes Research Institute would enforce the same rules requiring publication of positive and negative results that are now in effect for the clinicaltrials.gov website. Hernán voiced strong support for this idea, adding that selective reporting is a major problem for the field.

Mitchell H. Gail raised the point that RCTs themselves can be an important source of information on generalizability. He said that if an RCT finds that treatment effects are homogeneous throughout the study population, generalizability should be more straightforward and reweighting becomes simpler. Kaizar agreed with that statement but also said that too many studies make that leap without much evidence. Califf added that most every RCT shows effect heterogeneity across subgroups but that issues arise when attempts are made to generalize to populations far different from the trial population. He reminded the workshop participants that the majority of RCTs select more homogeneous trial populations to increase the odds that they will demonstrate a positive effect of the treatment, so the detection of subgroup heterogeneity within the trial population should not be surprising.

When asked by a workshop participant from a remote site about how to generalize treatment profiles in RCTs, Califf said that this is a big problem that the field needs to address. He cited as an example the Neonatal Intensive Care Unit Network Trial on the effects of oxygen saturation in neonates. The findings of this study were the opposite of those expected from observational studies, and a follow-up showed that mortality among neonates who were not enrolled in the study was higher even than that in the arm of the clinical trial with the worst mortality. One possibility is that whatever other treatments were being used outside of the RCT protocol were not only more variable but worse. Califf added that global trials on diet and medicinal herbs are extreme examples in which the variability in treatment profiles is so large as to be unmeasurable with current instruments.

Robert Temple noted that forest plots can provide a great deal of useful information about generalizability but that most reported studies on symptomatic treatments do not include them. He added that FDA is writing guidance that will encourage the use of forest plots and that will require demographic subset analysis.

Steven N. Goodman remarked that most of the work on heterogeneity and extrapolation that has been done has focused on the benefits of treatment but not the potential harms. Because most people want to know both the benefits and harms of any potential treatment that they might undergo, the issue of absolute versus relative risk becomes important. In that case, a therapy must surpass a higher standard, that is, whether it works well enough to overcome the potential harms and not just whether it works. In that regard, exclusion criteria in RCTs leave a large gap in the data because comorbidities are likely to play an important role in determining the risk of harm. Califf agreed with this point and noted that homogeneity often vanishes when one is looking at the benefit-to-risk ratio rather than just the benefits of treatment.

REFERENCES

Doyle, E. A., S. A. Weinzimer, A. T. Steffen, J. A. H. Ahern, M. Vincent, and W. V. Tamborlane. 2004. A randomized, prospective trial comparing the efficacy of continuous subcutaneous insulin infusion with multiple daily injections using insulin glargine. *Diabetes Care* 27:1554–1558.

Greenhouse, J. B., E. E. Kaizar, K. Kelleher, H. Seltman, and W. Gardner. 2008. Generalizing from clinical trial data: A case study. The risk of suicidality among pediatric antidepressant users. *Statistics in Medicine* 27(11):1801–1813.

Hernán, M. A., A. Alonso, R. Logan, F. Grodstein, K. B. Michels, W. C. Willett, J. E. Manson, and J. M. Robins. 2008. Observational studies analyzed like randomized experiments: An application to postmenopausal hormone therapy and coronary heart disease. *Epidemiology* 19(6):766–779.

Manson, J. E., J. Hsia, K. C. Johnson, J. E. Rossouw, A. R. Assaf, N. L. Lasser, M. Trevisan, H. R. Black, S. R. Heckbert, R. Detrano, O. L. Strickland, N. D. Wong, J. R. Crouse, E. Stein, M. Cushman, and the Women's Health Initiative Investigators. 2003. Estrogen plus progestin and the risk of coronary heart disease. *New England Journal of Medicine* 349(6):523–534.

Stampfer, M. J., and G. A. Colditz. 1991. Estrogen replacement therapy and coronary heart disease: A quantitative assessment of the epidemiologic evidence. *Preventative Medicine* 20(1):47–63.

U.S. General Accounting Office. 1992. *Cross-Design Synthesis: A New Strategy for Medical Effectiveness Research.* Report GAO/PEMD-92-18. Washington, DC: U.S. General Accounting Office. http://archive.gao.gov/d31t10/145906.pdf (accessed May 16, 2013).

Wallentin, L., R. C. Becker, A. Budaj, C. P. Cannon, H. Emanuelsson, C. Held, J. Horrow, S. Husted, S. James, H. Katus, K. W. Mahaffey, B. M. Scirica, A. Skene, P. G. Steg, R. F. Storey, and R. A. Harrington for the PLATO Investigators. 2009. Ticagrelor versus Clopidogrel in Patients with Acute Coronary Syndromes. *New England Journal of Medicine* 361:1045–1057.

Weintraub, W. S., M. V. Grau-Sepulveda, J. M. Weiss, S. M. O'Brien, E. D. Peterson, P. Kolm, Z. Zhang, L. W. Klein, R. E. Shaw, C. McKay, L. L. Ritzenhaler, J. J. Popma, J. C. Messenger, D. M. Shahian, F. L. Grover, J. E. Mayer, C. M. Shewan, K. N. Garratt, I. D. Moussa, G. D. Dangas, and F. H. Edwards. 2012. Comparative effectiveness of revascularization strategies. *New England Journal of Medicine* 366(16):1467–1476.

5

Detecting Treatment-Effect Heterogeneity

KEY SPEAKER THEMES

Kent

- Heterogeneity in treatment effects is likely to be ubiquitous, and the failure to detect it represents a failure of science.
- Hidden heterogeneity often leads to misleading results from randomized controlled trials (RCTs), but current approaches to subgroup analysis of clinical trials are inadequate and can be misleading.

Hlatky

- Pooling of data from multiple RCTs can identify effect heterogeneity, but subgroups can still be too small to generate statistically significant differences.
- Well-planned observational studies conducted to answer specific questions with data from large databases can identify heterogeneity in treatment effects and enable individualized recommendations.

Basu

- Individual patient differences are of crucial importance, and the study of heterogeneity over broad subgroups may not be useful in comparative effectiveness research.
- Algorithmic predictions generated from large observational data sets and then validated in confirmatory studies may be a promising way to guide clinical decision making.
- Methods to generate individual-level predictions from large observational studies must deal with the causal inference problems of such data. Newer instrumental variable methods are being developed to address these issues.

Moderator Richard Platt, chair of ambulatory care and prevention and chair of population medicine at Harvard University, introduced this session by noting that its focus on treatment subgroups was a fitting end to a day of discussions that highlighted the importance of sorting out treatment effects on subgroups in observational studies and randomized controlled trials (RCTs). Toward that end, David M. Kent, director of the Clinical and Translational Science Program at the Tufts University Sackler School of Graduate Biomedical Sciences, presented an overview on the detection of heterogeneity in treatment effects; Mark A. Hlatky discussed a specific example in which heterogeneity in treatment effects was observed in RCTs and observational studies; and Anirban Basu, associate professor and director of the Program in Health Economics and Outcomes Methodology at the University of Washington, spoke about the use of instrumental variables to identify heterogeneity in treatment effects. Mary E. Charlson, chief of clinical epidemiology and evaluative sciences research at Weill Cornell Medical College, and Mark R. Cullen, professor of medicine at the Stanford School of Medicine, commented on the presentations before the floor was opened for discussion.

KEY CONCEPTS IN HETEROGENEITY

The first concept that David M. Kent discussed was the fallacy of division, an idea that says that it is dangerous to make inferences about individuals or subgroups from aggregate results. He acknowledged, though, that evidence-based medicine, by necessity, is based largely on the making of such inferences. "We take group data, we measure treatment effects, and then we make inferences to the individuals in that group," he said. He explained that individual treatment effects are, generally, inherently unobservable because it is impossible to measure the outcome in an individual patient simultaneously both on and off treatment. Instead, clinical trials study a group of patients that receive treatment and a matched group that does not, measure the outcomes in those two groups, and then determine the benefit by comparing the proportion of patients in each group with a particular outcome. The treatment effect summarizing the difference in outcomes between the groups is then described in a probabilistic or stochastic manner and applied back to individuals.

Heterogeneity in treatment effects, in Kent's mind, is ubiquitous, and the failure to detect it represents a failure of science. Although he conceded that this is not a universally accepted idea, he said that it is consistent with the available evidence. Failure to detect heterogeneity even in the presence of marked differences in treatment effects across individuals can occur for myriad reasons. For example, observable covariates may be totally unrelated to the causal determinants of variations in treatment effects, or the causal mechanisms may be so complex that it is difficult to distinguish these from process statistical noise.

More potentially addressable problems include the limitations of the current analytical approach to subgroup analysis. For example, the statistical power to detect heterogeneity in the expected treatment effect is typically woefully inadequate when studies are powered to detect an overall treatment benefit. Analytic failure can also result from a limitation of conventional subgroup analysis, what Kent calls the "one-variable-at-a-time approach" to subgroup analysis. This type of subgroup analysis—for example, of males versus females or diabetics versus nondiabetics—is convenient but artificial because real patients simultaneously differ on multiple variables. As a result, the individuals in these one-variable-at-a-time subgroup analyses do not represent the full heterogeneity of patients that might be relevant for measurement of heterogeneous treatment effects that may be detected when combinations of variables are used (such as when multivariate risk models are employed).

Hidden heterogeneity often leads to misleading results from RCTs, said Kent in summary, but subgroup analysis of clinical trials is inadequate (because it is typically underpowered) and can also be misleading (because it is prone to spurious false-positive results). Despite voicing this negative outlook on treatment effect heterogeneity, Kent recommended three steps that could be taken to at least partially address some of these issues. First, investigators need to limit the number of hypothesis-testing subgroup analyses that they perform. One approach that may be used to do this is to explicitly specify which analyses are primary. Such analyses include those few analyses that are supported by strong prior evidence and that are clinically actionable. Any other subgroup analyses, said Kent, should be explicitly labeled as exploratory. Such analyses are meant not to inform clinical practice but to inform future research. The second step investigators need to take is to increase the power of their studies, and third, they must replicate and confirm subgroup analyses when they do identify a meaningful heterogeneous treatment effect. The last two steps require reengineering of the clinical enterprise to enable much larger studies and might require a greater reliance on observational studies.

EXAMPLE OF COMPARATIVE EFFECTIVENESS

Each year, more than 1 million coronary revascularization procedures are performed worldwide, said Mark A. Hlatky, in explaining his interest in comparing two such procedures. Angioplasty, or percutaneous coronary intervention (PCI), is most often used for single-vessel disease, whereas the far more invasive coronary artery bypass grafting (CABG) is used for extensive triple-vessel disease. Either procedure is feasible for treating midseverity coronary artery disease, yet, despite the commonness of these procedures, their effects on mortality are uncertain. The two procedures have been compared in RCTs and observational studies, but these studies have focused on the general population and do not provide much guidance for specific patients. Hlatky noted that one of the early trials comparing the two procedures—the Bypass Angioplasty Revascularization Investigation trial in diabetics—did provide some evidence of a heterogeneous treatment effect. This was a controversial finding that was followed up in a number of studies, but all suffered from the concern that they were post hoc analyses that were, as he put it, "big fishing expeditions."

If RCTs are the preferred approach to comparing PCI with CABG but the trials are large enough only to examine the main effect, one way to look for heterogeneity in treatment effects is to pool together several RCTs and test whether the answer lies in a larger sample size. Hlatky and his collaborators did just that, organizing a collaboration of 10 randomized trials of bypass surgery and angioplasty and convincing the investigators to share data, which he noted is more of a political than a technical challenge. In the end, the resulting dataset included almost 8,000 patients and 1,200 deaths, and the data did reveal some treatment effect heterogeneity, which Hlatky illustrated using a forest plot (see Figure 5-1).

He explained that in the youngest patients in the trials, PCI produced better outcomes, whereas bypass surgery produced better outcomes in the oldest patients. The data confirmed that diabetes was a strong modifier of risk and that age also modified comparative effectiveness. Additional subgroups showed evidence of heterogeneous treatment effects, but too few of the enrolled subjects fell into these subgroups to produce statistically significant differences. The latter finding is not surprising, he said, because the selection criteria for most RCTs limit generalization by excluding comorbidities. Another factor that worked against generalization was that

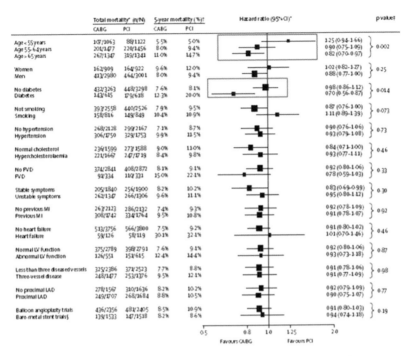

FIGURE 5-1 Outcomes in subgroups from 10 randomized clinical trials comparing coronary artery bypass grafting (CABG) and percutaneous coronary intervention (PCI).
SOURCE: Hlatky et al., 2009.

these trials were run at large medical centers with highly skilled staff, and the results may not represent those obtained by physicians in other clinical settings.

To address some of these limitations, Hlatky and his collaborators examined observational data to see if they could replicate and extend the findings from their pooled RCT study (Hlatky et al., 2013). They used the 20 percent Medicare sample from 1992 to 2008 to identify patients who were 66 years of age or older, which gave them at least 1 year to document comorbidities; received fee-for-service coverage, which yielded billing codes; and who underwent multivessel PCI or CABG. Hlatky and his colleagues used propensity score matching but also forced matches on the year in which patients received their treatment, whether they had diabetes, and their age within a year. The last step was taken because of suspected secular effects in the outcomes related to the year that the procedure was done. Each arm of the study had 105,000 patients. Treatment-covariate interactions were prespecified to produce relative differences, or hazard ratios, and absolute differences in terms of 5-year survival and the number of years of life added. The goal was to produce information that was actionable for patients.

The main findings of this study were that those who underwent CABG had lower mortality overall and a higher 5-year survival rate. Diabetes, heart failure, peripheral artery disease, and tobacco use all produced a significant modification of the treatment effect; and treatment effectiveness varied substantially. In fact, the analysis predicted that 41 percent of the population would have better survival if they underwent angioplasty, even though the overall result showed that CABG was superior in terms of mortality. This analysis demonstrated that a substantial heterogeneity in treatment effect could affect people's decision making, said Hlatky, and that seven patient variables could be used together to make individual predictions. He and his collaborators used these findings to create a coronary heart disease procedure calculator that could input a variety of patient characteristics—age, gender, tobacco use, prior hospitalization for a heart attack, diabetes, peripheral artery disease, and heart failure—and make an individual projection on which procedure would produce a higher 5-year survival, the range of the increased risk of mortality in similar patients, and the benefit in terms of longer life expectancy.

Hlatky closed his presentation by reflecting on the pooled RCT data and observational analyses he described, and stating that he was reassured by the fact that both found evidence of heterogeneity of treatment effectiveness. Finally, he called for the need to refocus efforts from focusing on overall effects to better detecting and understanding heterogeneity.

IDENTIFICATION OF EFFECT-HETEROGENEITY USING INSTRUMENTAL VARIABLES

Anirban Basu noted that the focus of his work is on effect heterogeneity and not response heterogeneity, which he said is an important distinction to make. "We are really interested in how much the incremental outcome between two treatments varies across people," he explained. As a recap of the day's earlier presentation on instrumental variables, he reminded the workshop participants that instrumental variables are those that influence treatment choices but that are independent of factors that determine potential outcomes, that they are viewed as natural randomizers, and that they can be used to establish the causal effects of a treatment by accounting for both overt and hidden biases.

Before discussing his own work, he described one classic example of the use of instrumental variables. In that study, the investigators used Medicare data to examine the effect of invasive cardiac treatment on long-term mortality rates (Stukel et al., 2007). The observed confounders were those typically found in Medicare data—age, sex, race, socioeconomic status, comorbidities, and inpatient treatment—and the unobserved confounder was the risk for the patient. Basu explained that the investigators were concerned that only low-risk patients were given invasive cardiac treatment, potentially leading to better outcomes from invasive treatments. With adjustment for differences in risk through the use of the propensity score or regression analysis, they found a huge positive effect of invasive cardiac treatment. However, when they repeated the analysis using the regional catheterization rate as the instrument variable, the effect was not as substantial when they adjusted for the selection of lower-risk patients for invasive cardiac treatment.

Building on that example, Basu discussed one approach to interpreting the results of an instrumental variable analysis when there is treatment effect heterogeneity. In the presence of heterogeneity in the treatment effect, there is no reason to believe that the causal effect of a treatment that comes out of an observational study should be the same as the causal effect of a treatment that comes out of an RCT, that the average treatment effect is a relevant metric for evaluation, or that the effect of the instrumental variable has a relevant interpretation. The first step in addressing these issues is to develop a choice model that starts with the assumption that the choice of treatment is based on an underlying latent index; the latent index is a function of observed confounders and instrumental variables, as well as a function of unobserved confounders and stochastic error. If the latent index is greater than zero, people choose to get treatment, and if it is less than zero, they do not choose to get treatment. This notion of an underlying latent index is pervasive today across choice models used in both statistics and econometrics, explained Basu. He also said that use of this type of model provides a good picture of who and who is not selecting treatment and how a treatment effect happens when instrumental variables exist.

By use of this simple model construct, instrumental variable methods estimate treatment effect by comparison of a group of people with some level of the instrumental variable with another group of people with a different level of the instrumental variable, with all observed characteristics kept constant. The difference in outcomes between those who choose treatment and those who do not, then yields an estimate of the treatment effect only for those groups of people whose treatment choice changes because of changes in the values of instrument. However, if the treatment effects are heterogeneous, then this treatment effect from the instrumental variable is conditional on the unobserved level of confounders, a fact that is sometimes called "essential heterogeneity" (Heckman and Vytlacil, 1999). A newer method, called the "local instrumental variable," provides a way around essential heterogeneity. What the local instrumental variable does, explained Basu, is to help identify the marginal treatment effects or the treatment effect for the person who is at the margin of choice defined by the choice model.

Once the marginal treatment effect is estimated, it is possible to determine a marginal treatment effect conditioned on various levels of observed and unobserved characteristics and to then aggregate across various populations to determine the average treatment effect and to extend that to a person-centered treatment effect. To illustrate one application of this approach, Basu discussed how he applied it using Medicaid data to compare the treatment effect of older, generic antipsychotic drugs and newer so-called atypical antipsychotics. The original Clinical Antipsychotic Trials of Intervention Effectiveness study funded by the National Institute of Mental Health found similar effectiveness between the two classes of drugs over an 18-month period (Lieberman et al., 2005). As a result, 40 percent of state-run Medicaid programs have instituted prior authorization restrictions on some atypical antipsychotic drugs, which may have played a role in the waning commitment by pharmaceutical companies to develop new drugs in the area of neuroscience.

Basu's analysis of Medicaid data showed a tremendous treatment heterogeneity that could not be explained by one covariate. This analysis showed that when patients received optimal therapy, in comparison with the status quo, the average number of hospitalizations in the 12 months following the initiation of atypical antipsychotic therapy was predicted to be nearly 28 percent lower. He concluded his remarks by noting that differences between individual patients are of crucial importance and that the study of heterogeneity over broad subgroups may not be useful in comparative effectiveness research. He also noted that the use of algorithmic predictions generated from large sets of data from observational studies and then validated in confirmatory studies may be a promising way to guide clinical decision making.

COMMENT

Heterogeneity is something that the field needs to stop running from, said Mary E. Charlson in commenting on the two presentations. Investigators have become too focused on standardization and uniformity, but this focus "leads us away from really doing the investigation of treatment heterogeneity response that I think can inform the next series of questions about what is working for patients and what is not." For example, she suggested that a closer examination of the baseline variables in the studies discussed by Hlatky might reveal that important aspects of the patients' experiences during and after the CABG or PCI procedures could be driving overall differences in mortality. She indicated that her work has found that patients who undergo CABG make important secondary lifestyle changes that likely have an impact on mortality, whereas the vast majority of PCI patients do not. She said that investigation of drivers of variability or heterogeneity in the treatment response helps expand the ability to help patients and improve the prognostic armamentarium.

Charlson called for the field to look at variables beyond those typically studied, such as depression and social isolation, and to expand the ability to collect data from patients directly through the use of modern technologies and techniques, such as crowd sourcing. She noted that patients are already sharing their experiences on social media sites and believed that collection of those stories, along with some quantitative data, could shape how the heterogeneity in the treatment response is studied. The capture of this kind of information is a major opportunity to learn more about actual patient experiences and outcomes and to customize how to better inform patients about which treatments are right for them.

Mark R. Cullen, whose background is in the study of the upstream causes of morbidity and mortality in the workplace, said that the workplace is an interesting and challenging environment in which to study heterogeneity in treatment effects for at least three reasons. First, all studies must be observational, because RCTs would be impractical and unethical in the workplace environment. Second, extraordinary and conspicuous selection pressures exist in the populations coming into and going out of the workplace. The quantification and management of these pressures are methodologically problematic, but such pressures are highly visible in ways that confounders at the bedside are not. Third, substantial heterogeneity exists in the way in which people respond to adverse physical elements in the workplace environment.

With that as background, Cullen said that it was surprising that the field has not developed a simplifying rule for model making that breaks down questions into those that involve a treatment choice at a single point in time. From that choice made at a single point in time, it would then be possible to develop a marginal structural model to deal with the changes that occur over the course of observation. He agreed with Miguel A. Hernán's view, presented in the prior session, that observational research and RCTs have a great deal in common and that one of the major issues in working in the observational domain is where and how to use instrumental variables or other strategies to effectively randomize the environment in which randomization is not occurring.

Cullen noted that the field needs a new way to look at studies of large populations. "We have bought in to a very stochastic way of looking at questions of whether something has efficacy that is based on a certain set of assumptions," he said. "We are averaging over all kinds of different effects and are imagining that those effects are in essence random." In contrast, he noted, "many of our colleagues not represented here do not take that view at all, but live in a very deterministic world in which they would imagine the only thing interesting about heterogeneity is how much we do or do not know about the underlying biology." As an example, he cited the situation in the cancer world, in which breast cancer is no longer treated as one heterogeneous disease but as distinctly different diseases based on the underlying biology. This will play out in a way in which these biological discriminators are not likely to fall into the categories now used to explain heterogeneity, such as race, sex, and age. He thought that one area in which this type of heterogeneity could begin to be evaluated would be in individuals with unique, preexisting diseases.

He concluded his remarks by discussing how the combined use of a propensity score type of approach and an instrumental variable might be useful for examining heterogeneity. In a study of neonatal intensive care units at two hospitals, one of Cullen's students used proximity to the unit as the instrumental variable and formed matched pairs that were identical on everything observable except for distance from the neonatal intensive care unit. From this subset of individuals, the student was able to define the enormous benefit for mortality for infants at one hospital over mortality for infants at the other. This student is now looking at subgroups to see if differences with sufficient power to draw conclusions about a particular subset of high-risk mothers or high-risk infants exist. The beauty of this approach, said Cullen, is how simple it is to do this kind of analysis.

DISCUSSION

Platt said he was impressed that all five speakers were to some degree sanguine about the prospects for doing subgroup analysis. A workshop participant then remarked that to him, the idea of creating risk models to create subgroups or models that identify those who may have different absolute reductions in risk from a treatment is a good one but that it is not the right approach for finding factors that could modify the treatment effect, particularly biological risk factors. Instead, the use of actual biological modifiers rather than risk models should be the more appropriate approach. He encouraged the field to think hard about how the biology works and create subgroups that are not based on risk models but that are based on models of how the biology might be modified by those factors.

Another participant said that he would like to see forest plots created according to absolute rather than relative risk reduction. He also commented that many physicians ignore the findings of RCTs because of the population that was tested. He cited two examples: gynecologists who say that the findings from the Women's Health Initiative study on hormone replacement therapy do not apply to their patients who are younger than age 60 years and orthopedic surgeons who still perform vertebroplasty, despite the data from a high-quality trial showing that this procedure does not benefit patients.

A participant commented that the talks so far failed to make a connection between observational studies and what they can bring to a learning health care system and suggested that the Institute of Medicine hold another meeting to deal explicitly with that connection. The same participant also wondered how to take the heterogeneity of the effectiveness of an intervention being measured and use that to study what are inherently complex, multiattribute decisions. He questioned, too, whether many examples of a treatment demonstrating efficacy in an RCT but not being effective when used correctly really exist.

The same participant wondered if data heterogeneity is being swamped by the heterogeneity of medical practice and patient preferences. Basu and Charlson thought that might be the case but that good opportunities to learn from those individual patient experiences exist and that this knowledge may inform a learning health care system. Charlson reiterated her earlier proposal that the field needs to develop methods to more systematically capture individual patient experiences beyond those recorded in electronic health records. Sheldon Greenfield agreed with this proposal because he believes that many of the variables related to heterogeneity that are now considered unobservable would be observable if both patients and physicians were queried more systematically. Hlatky agreed with these recommendations but cautioned that the solution does not always lie in more data; it lies in only more good-quality data.

Marc L. Berger asked the panelists if there were opportunities for examining heterogeneity in Phase II studies and generating hypotheses that could be examined in Phase III studies as a way of improving the productivity of the drug development pipeline. Basu replied that the only way to do that is to greatly expand the number of subgroups—and the budget—for Phase II trials. Charlson said that the field needs to look more carefully at adaptive clinical trial designs. Joe V. Selby noted that this would be a good topic for another workshop.

In response to a question about whether the subgroups in his studies were based at all on biology, Hlatky responded that they were not and that it would be interesting to look for biological correlates to the subgroup classifiers. Cullen pointed out that the subgroup classifiers that Hlatky and his colleagues identified are the ones that surgeons are most likely to use to make real therapeutic decisions when facing a patient. Hlatky added that in the case of cardiac surgery, certain psychosocial factors that are not biological play major roles in the outcome.

Steven N. Goodman remarked that he had not heard anyone address the subject of multiplicity, which he said will become important with the advent of massive databases containing biological data from genomics, proteomics, and other -omics and data-mining tools that will generate what he said will effectively be an infinite number of subgroups. "I am definitely not a zealot about correcting for the multiplicity," he said, "but it reflects in some ways indirectly our lack of understanding of biologic processes [in our] explanations. It is something we cannot ignore."

REFERENCES

Heckman, J. J., and E. J. Vytlacil. 1999. Local instrumental variables and latent variable models for identifying and bounding treatment effects. *Proceedings of the National Academy of Sciences of the United States of America* 96(8):4730–4734.

Hlatky, M. A., D. B. Boothroyd, D. M. Bravata, E. Boersma, J. Booth, M. M. Brooks, D. Carrié, T. C. Clayton, N. Danchin, M. Flather, C. W. Hamm, W. A. Hueb, J. Kähler, S. F. Kelsey, S. B. King, A. S. Kosinski, N. Lopes, K. M. McDonald, A. Rodriguez, P. Serruys, U. Sigwart, R. H. Stables, D. K. Owens, and S. J. Pocock. 2009. Coronary artery bypass surgery compared with percutaneous coronary interventions for multivessel disease: A collaborative analysis of individual patient data from ten randomised trials. *Lancet* 373(9670):1190–1197.

Hlatky, M. A., D. B. Boothroyd, L. Baker, D. S. Kazi, M. D. Solomon, T. I. Chang, D. Shilane, and A. S. Go. 2013. Comparative effectiveness of multivessel coronary bypass surgery and multivessel percutaneous coronary intervention: A cohort study. *Annals of Internal Medicine* 158(10):727–734.

Lieberman, J. A., T. S. Stroup, J. P. McEvoy, M. S. Swartz, R. A. Rosenheck, D. O. Perkins, R. S. E. Keefe, S. M. Davis, C. E. Davis, B. D. Lebowitz, J. Severe, and J. K. Hsiao for the Clinical Antipsychotic Trials of Intervention Effectiveness (CATIE) Investigators. 2005. Effectiveness of Antipsychotic Drugs in Patients with Chronic Schizophrenia. *New England Journal of Medicine* 353:1209–1223.

Stukel, T. A., E. S. Fisher, D. E. Wennberg, D. A. Alter, D. J. Gottlieb, and M. J. Vermeulen. 2007. Analysis of observational studies in the presence of treatment selection bias: Effects of invasive cardiac management on AMI survival using propensity score and instrumental variable methods. *Journal of the American Medical Association* 297(3):278–285.

6

Predicting Individual Responses

KEY SPEAKER THEMES

Singer

- Although issues concerning study design are important, the field of clinical research also needs to start considering methods with the goal of enabling physician inquiries.
- The Patient-Centered Outcomes Research Institute should promote the development of strategies to allow for approximate matching of individual patients with records of similar patients and then conduct tests to see what happens when physicians make treatment decisions using these strategies.

Tatonetti

- Propensity score matching can be used to correct for the effects of bias of measured covariates in observational studies. However, this requires having measurements for all confounding variables, which is rarely the case.
- Implicit propensity score matching can be used to overcome limitations related to sparse information on confounders in databases of spontaneous reports of drug adverse events.

Kattan

- The diagnostic gestalt is overrated because each physician has too many biases and too many variables to accurately compute therapeutic outcome probabilities.
- Data from electronic health records, although imperfect, yield reasonably accurate statistical prediction models that are often better than those based on the simple staging strategies currently used to predict risk.

The bottom line for medical decision making is to develop a course of therapy that will provide the greatest benefit to an individual patient with the lowest chance of harm. In this session, three speakers and two additional panelists discussed the challenges with the use of data from groups of individuals from randomized controlled trials (RCTs) and observational studies to guide treatment choices for specific individuals. Burton H. Singer, professor at the Emerging Pathogens Institute at the University of Florida, provided a short introduction to the subject. Nicholas Tatonetti, assistant professor of biomedical informatics at Colombia University, described the use of data-driven prediction models, and Michael W. Kattan, chair of the Quantitative Health Sciences Department at the Cleveland Clinic, described one method of predicting individual risk from treatment. Mitchell H. Gail and Peter Bach, an attending physician in the Department of Epidemiology and Biostatistics at the Memorial Sloan-Kettering Cancer Center, commented on the two presentations before an open discussion period.

INTRODUCTION TO INDIVIDUAL RESPONSE PREDICTION

Burton H. Singer asked the workshop to put aside for the moment thinking about study design, which was such an important focus of the previous day's discussions, and instead consider the concept of inquiry. Consider a clinician talking to a patient, he said. In front of this physician is an elaborate patient record that includes biomarker information; notes about the patient's experiences in care, such as the ones that Mary E. Charlson emphasized; a clinical history; and perhaps a history of the patient's psychosocial well-being. Having read and absorbed all of that information, the clinician's job at that moment is to determine the likely performance of a contemplated treatment regimen for the patient. Singer stressed the word "regimen," because this treatment will not be an activity that takes places at just one point in time but is one that will occur over time. It is right then, at that moment, that the physician wants to conduct an inquiry, not a study.

What the physician wants at that moment is access to a large database that he or she can query to find patients who are approximate matches to the patient sitting across the desk. These approximate matches would not be matches just on particular variables but, rather, would be matches on an entire history as the unit of analysis, which would be characterized by a description of the patient's condition at multiple time points. Next, the physician would query the database to identify the experiences that these approximate matches have had with the intended treatment regimen and compare them with the experiences that others have had. With that information in hand, the physician could then talk to his or her patient about the potential benefits and risks of the planned treatment in the context of what others with similar disease and personal characteristics have experienced. All of this, said Singer, presumes that the database is populated with high-quality data.

To reach this ideal state of medical practice, the Patient-Centered Outcomes Research Institute (PCORI) should promote an effort to develop approximate matching strategies and then conduct tests to see what happens when physicians make treatment decisions using these strategies. Singer noted that heterogeneity among both patients and physician practice will play a large role in this effort. For physicians, heterogeneity will show itself in terms of the types of treatments that they use and how they react to and use the answers to their queries: will they take the advice from the database query, ignore it, or modify it in some way? He acknowledged the substantial methodological challenge in accounting for physician-associated heterogeneity but suggested that these challenges can be tackled first by evaluation of individual disease processes.

He concluded his presentation with a quote from a 1977 paper published in *Science* by John Tukey, who wrote:

> It is a difficult task to drive the nearly incompatible two-horse team: on the one hand, knowledge of a most carefully evaluated kind, where, in particular, questions of multiplicity are faced up to; and, on the other, informed professional opinion, where impressions gained from statistically inadequate numbers of cases often, and so far as we see, often should, control the treatment of individual patients. The same physician or surgeon must be concerned with both what is his knowledge and what is his informed professional opinion, often as part of treating a single patient. I wish I understood better how to help in this essentially ambivalent task.

Singer said that in his mind this statement is still relevant today and that part of PCORI's mission should be to address the issues that the statement raises by thinking about clinical inquiry as a part of making individualized predictions.

DATA-DRIVEN PREDICTION MODELS

Nicholas Tatonetti noted in his opening remarks that his presentation was not going to be directly applicable to the prediction of individualized responses but that the methodologies that he would be discussing represent the first step in that direction. With that as a caveat, he said that one of his interests is in drug safety, and he spoke about the balance between the health benefits and risks associated with the small-molecule drugs that he characterized as the cornerstone of modern medical practice. Discussing the alert issued by the U.S. Food and Drug Administration (FDA) in 2012 for the statin family of cholesterol-controlling drugs, Tatonetti said that although statins are one of the safest groups of drugs known, even drugs considered safe and effective can unexpectedly cause dangerous side effects. He also reminded the workshop of Vioxx and Avandia, two drugs that were approved and later pulled from the market when reports of severe side effects with widespread use began appearing.

In the aftermath of the Vioxx and Avandia incidents, there was a public call for the establishment of a public database to monitor drug safety, but FDA has been maintaining such a database for more than 30 years as part of the Adverse Events Reporting System. Today, this database comprises more than 3 million reports, an enormous observational database, but it is of limited utility because it is only sparsely populated with data on patient age, sex, weight, and country; the drugs that a patient was taking at the time of the adverse event; or the conditions for which a patient was receiving treatment. As a result of the sparse information, these reports are hard to interpret, Tatonetti said, and in fact, such spontaneous reporting systems in general are biased and introduce "synthetic associations" in terms of concomitant drug use and indication. As an example of the former, he said that a naïve analysis of the FDA Adverse Event Report System or most any clinical observational dataset would reveal a connection between aspirin use and heart attack. However, a deeper assessment of the data in the dataset would show an enormous signal for Vioxx and heart attacks that creates a false association with other drugs coprescribed with Vioxx. As an example of an indication effect, he said drugs given to diabetics are more likely to be associated with hyperglycemia in the adverse report dataset, which he termed a nonsensical result, given that the real association is with poor control of diabetes and not a particular diabetes drug.

Propensity score matching, said Tatonetti, is a technique used with observational studies that corrects for these very types of effects arising from the bias of measured covariates. Use of this technique requires identification of matched controls for the studied cases and modeling of the likelihood that the patient is selected for inclusion in the study on the basis of covariates, which in this case would be drug exposure. This method produces effect estimates that are close to those seen in idealized RCTs, but its drawback is that it requires the availability of measurements for all confounding variables, which is rarely the case with spontaneously collected data.

To address this limitation, Tatonetti developed implicit propensity score matching (IPSM), an adapted form of propensity matching that assumes that combinations of drugs and indications describe the patient's covariates. Having a list of the drugs that a patient is taking can provide much information about a patient, he explained. This method starts with reports in the database that list both coprescribed prescriptions and significantly correlated indications, and this group of reports serves as the source of the matched controls. As an example, he discussed the nonsensical association that he had mentioned earlier between diabetes drugs and hyperglycemia. In the adverse events database, 17.7 percent of reports of diabetes drugs list hyperglycemia as an adverse event. If the entire database served as the control, approximately 1.5 percent of the reports would list hyperglycemia as an adverse event, producing the apparent association. However, if the control cohort is restricted by use of the IPSM technique, the frequency at which hyperglycemia would be an expected adverse event reported in association with all other drugs that a patient is taking would be 17.6 percent, revealing the false association with diabetes drugs.

He described another example in which IPSM corrects for the association between arrhythmia and antiarrhythmic drugs, in which 10 of 13 drugs identified without correction by the use of IPSM were no longer associated with what is known as the "prorhythmic effect." The three drugs whose proportional reporting ratio still exceeded the significance threshold after correction by the use of IPSM do, in fact, have prorhythmic effects that limit their use. IPSM, he added, can also correct for other biases, such as age or sex.

Another issue that this approach addresses is under- and nonreporting of adverse events. In this case, severe adverse events are identified by the presence of more minor—and more common—side effects. In essence, Tatonetti explained, this is much like the way in which a physician detects disease: the physician uses observable side effects to form a hypothesis about the underlying disease. In this case, the procedure first involves identification of common side effects that are harbingers for the underlying severe adverse event. These are then combined to form an effect profile for an adverse event.

As an example, he showed how IPSM was used with electronic health record (EHR) data to identify a drug-drug interaction between paroxetine and pravastatin, a combination that some 1 million patients take annually (Tatonetti et al., 2011). A previous observational study that used data from EHRs showed evidence of an interaction between these two drugs that resulted in increased blood glucose levels, but this study could have been biased by confounders, such as the use of other combinations of drugs in the paroxetine class and other statins, the time of day that glucose readings were taken, and the concomitant use of other medications. IPSM analysis found that none of these were significant confounders. Skeptics remained, however, so he and his collaborators ran a small experiment in mice and found virtually the same result seen in humans: the combination of paroxetine and pravastatin, particularly in insulin-resistant mice, produces a significant increase in blood glucose levels.

INDIVIDUALIZED PREDICTION OF RISK

Michael W. Kattan's interest in predicting personal risk began when his physician told him he had Stage IV Hodgkin's lymphoma. When he asked about his chances for surviving this disease, he was shown the typical prognostic plots, which were based solely on disease staging, and concluded that this particular counseling tool was not designed to predict his prognosis accurately. Kattan explained that when asked that question, physicians have two choices: either quote an overall average to all patients or make a prediction based on knowledge and experience. What the physician needs instead is some way of taking as many relevant pieces of information about a specific patient as possible and using that to inform a model to make a personalized prediction that informs therapeutic choices.

As an example of a simple model, he described a preoperative nomogram for prostate cancer that assigns point values for three characteristics—the prostate-specific antigen (PSA) level, the patient's clinical state, and the biopsy Gleason grade—and then relates the point total to the probability that the patient will be free of prostate cancer after 5 years (Kattan et al., 1998). This model can be modified to include risk stratification depending on surgery or radiation therapy and therefore inform a patient's decision on the basis of the risk of a 5-year recurrence with one type of therapy or the other. He showed a similar nomogram that was also better than simple staging at predicting the probability of 5-year survival for patients with gastric cancer. He concluded that on the basis of his experience, this type of continuous regression equation modeling produces at least a small amount of discrimination compared with that achieved with simple staging systems.

One problem that Kattan has noticed with these predictive tools is that surgeons are reluctant to use them. He recounted one study that he and his colleagues conducted in which they presented 10 case descriptions from real prostate cancer patients to 17 urologists. The urologists were provided with PSA, biopsy Gleason grades, clinical stage, patient age, systematic biopsy details, previous biopsy results, and PSA history. They were also provided with the preoperative nomogram and were asked to make their own predictions of the probability of 5-year progression-free cancer with or without the use of the nomogram. The results showed that concordance with the patient's actual 5-year survival was 67 percent with the nomogram, whereas it was 55 percent when the urologists made the prediction on the basis of experience (Ross et al., 2002). In a similar study in which a nomogram was used to predict the likelihood of additional nodal metastases in breast cancer patients with a positive sentinel node biopsy result, the nomogram was 72 percent accurate at making predictions, whereas clinicians were 54 percent accurate (Van Zee et al., 2003).

Based on these types of comparisons, Kattan concludes that the diagnostic gestalt is overrated because each physician has too many biases and the presence of too many variables makes it difficult to accurately compute the probabilities of various therapeutic outcomes. He indicated that he would like to see the field develop comparative effectiveness tables. He acknowledged that tailoring such tables to an individual is difficult, but he added, "I think efficiencies and better decision making would take place if we could get that type of information handed to us." He showed an example of a risk calculator developed at the Cleveland Clinic that uses its EHR to fill in an individual's information on age, gender, comorbid conditions, medications, blood pressure, lipid levels, smoking status, and other personal characteristics to produce a table that provides 6-year probabilities of mortality, stroke, coronary artery disease, liver injury, heart failure, renal insufficiency, and diabetic nephropathy for each of four classes of diabetes drugs (see Table 6-1).

After describing some of the programming that is needed to create these tools, he noted that the Cleveland Clinic has developed more than two

TABLE 6-1 Example Individualized Predictive Risks of Seven Outcomes Across Four Drugs Given to Diabetic Patients

OUTCOMES (6-year probabilities)	DRUG CLASS			
	BIG	MEG	SFU	TZD
Mortality	0.013	0.122	0.054	0.042
Stroke	0.016	0.021	0.018	0.016
Coronary Artery Disease	0.024	0.005	0.028	0.033
Livery Injury	0.073	0.114	0.105	0.089
Heart Failure	0.010	0.015	0.014	0.012
Renal Insufficiency	0.087	0.176	0.130	0.110
Diabetic Nephropathy	0.467	0.386	0.451	0.562

NOTE: BIG = biguanides; MEG = meglitinides; SFU = sulfonylurea; TZD = thiazolidinedione.
SOURCE: Reprinted with permission from Michael W. Kattan.

dozen of these risk calculators that input patient EHR data; the calculators are available to the public at http://rcalc.ccf.org. Also available is a tool for constructing new risk calculators that anyone is free to use with registration. In conclusion, he said that data from EHRs, although imperfect, yield reasonably accurate statistical prediction models, though many modeling options should be compared to determine their predictive accuracies. He added that the collection of follow-up data is the biggest challenge with verification of the accuracy of these models.

COMMENT

In his comments, Mitchell H. Gail noted that the concept of matching that Singer described had been widely used since the 1800s, until the RCT was introduced. He said that it has been argued that databases can address a wider range of questions than can RCTs but that is true only if the right things can be matched in a way that controls confounding by indication. As an example, he cited work done in the 1980s on thyroid cancer that showed that patients who received radiation therapy did far worse than those who had surgery, but the study could not conclude that radiation was the problem because the registry contained no information in indicating why the patient received radiation instead of surgery.

He then commended Tatonetti for his assessment of how observational data from large data sets can be used to identify adverse events. This approach to controlling for confounding by indication was interesting, but he took a wait-and-see attitude as to whether this method works, pending further studies to gain more experience with IPSM. Gail agreed with Kattan's assessment about the need for highly discriminating and well-calibrated risk models, but he said that the approach that he took in his work avoided the question of confounding by indication.

Peter Bach agreed with Gail that the issue of confounding is important, as are concerns about the quality of the data in large data sets. He said that one of the challenges that the field faces today is the tension between the use of ever larger data sets and not being able to overcome some of the intrinsic, unmeasured differences between groups. In fact, he said that he worries that "the illusion of precise information could actually move us in the wrong direction." As an example, he cited a seeming 10-fold difference in mortality that appeared in the diabetes table that Kattan presented. "It seems inconceivable to me that a single drug could drive that kind of mortality difference. But certainly, if I saw it as a patient and believed the numbers in front of me, it would certainly heavily influence my decision-making process," he explained.

The issue of collecting follow-up data is an important problem, Bach continued. In the cancer world, for example, although the time and cause of death are relatively easy to obtain, data on progression and time to progression are difficult to capture because patients move around and because they are actually heavily influenced by surveillance schedules and other aspects of treatment that are in themselves confounded. He then discussed work on lung cancer screening that showed the power of these predictive models to identify people at risk for interventions and counsel patients about the benefits and risks. He also remarked that the field needs to do more work on risk communication both to promote more research in the area and to help patients use available tools.

DISCUSSION

William S. Weintraub raised the issue of confounding by indication and remarked how none of the different risk models that could be developed using observational studies and RCTs fully address this issue. He asked members of the panel for their thoughts on two questions: How should the field go forward in developing good risk models? What are the best methods of assessing the quality of a given risk model? Responding to the first question, Kattan agreed that confounding by indication is a tough problem to solve. He said that RCTs could provide the best solutions but that in the cardiac field, surgeons and radiologists would never allow the kinds of trial designs that would answer questions regarding confounding by indication. Tatonetti agreed that RCTs are the preferred source of risk data but that they become infeasible when drug-drug interactions or comorbidity effects are being studied. "The number of patients you need is simply too large and the costs are too large, so these technologies need to be investigated," said Tatonetti. "The problem is, we do not have a lot of validation that they produce reliable effect risk estimates."

Horwitz asked the panel if the current risk models are providing data that may be misleading patients when they make decisions. Kattan replied that it was possible but added that the current models may still be providing information better than that which one would have if no models were available. Tatonetti said that his is a data-mining method and that it is not designed for developing a precise risk model in any one setting. "I would not be confident enough that I corrected for confounding so well that I would trust the risk estimates that come out of it," said Tatonetti, adding that rather than trying to correct for confounding, he tries to corroborate the results with those from another dataset. "I think that is essential, especially when you are using these confounded observational data sets to continue to try and find a complementary dataset that has slightly different information and slightly different biases and you can start to build up a kind of corpus of evidence that suggests that maybe your hypothesis is true."

Gail noted that "there are books written on the best way to formulate models and on the criteria for evaluating them, and I think very well established ways of checking how well calibrated a model is. So I think some of the technical aspects of modeling have received a lot of attention and are continuing to receive attention, but there are adequate methods." He agreed with Bach that observational data can add to the estimation of risk in a way that is meaningful to the patient, particularly because the trial population in an RCT can be too small to provide reliable baseline estimates of absolute risk.

Michael Pencina, associate professor in the Department of Mathematics and Statistics at Boston University, remarked that he considers website prediction models such as the ones that Kattan described to be controversial. "We have a lot of them, but very few have been validated," he said, noting that he has had discussions with the FDA regarding whether the agency should be monitoring this activity and to what extent. The big question, he said, is how to validate these models. "My answer is [that] it almost does not matter which metric we use to assess model performance as [much as] it does whether we understand what they tell us and what the standards are for interpretation," said Pencina. In other words, he added, "What is good enough?" Kattan agreed with this critique of Web-based models for public use and said that he and his colleagues do not post a prediction tool until they are comfortable with the foundational procedures and the error measures. He thought that, ideally, all such tools should have a link to a publication that a physician can access before recommending the tool to a patient.

David M. Kent, commenting on Kattan's use of risk models in concert with clinical trials, said that his research has been finding what he called a surprising degree of risk variation even in efficacy trials and that the typical patient typically has a much lower risk than the summary effect in the overall trial results. He also noted that although Kattan's work showed that the gestalt of physicians often does not agree with the actual risk, prediction models often disagree with one another as well and produce different recommendations. In response, Bach said that it is vitally important to understand the user of these predictions and thought that this was an area ripe for study, in particular, how doctors comprehend risk prediction.

Sanford Schwartz, professor of internal medicine, health care management, economics, and medicine at the University of Pennsylvania, said that it is important to identify the clinical objective before a model is designed. "Is the objective to identify risk?" he asked. "Is it to inform the doctor and the patient about alternative trade-offs of prognosis or alternative trade-offs of treatment?" It is more important, he said, to consider clinical utility than absolute accuracy, particularly in the context of advising patients in a learning health system and what PCORI is trying to accomplish in that context. In his mind, the risk and health care costs of a false-positive result versus a false-negative result may be a greater for one application, but the opposite could be true for another application.

Providing feedback for PCORI, Schwartz said that observational studies are going to be critically important because RCTs can look at only a subset of outcomes and not the range of outcomes that are important to doctors and patients. The key, he said, is to fill in missing data, and he recommended that PCORI focus on "trying to generate registries or observational data sets where there is an emphasis on follow-up, on getting [data about] what happens to the person longitudinally." He added that PCORI should also focus on developing ways for presenting information to doctors and patients and on understanding how that information will be interpreted by patients and physicians.

In response to a question from Horwitz about what needs to be done to provide predictions that reflect longitudinal changes in treatment, condition, or comorbidities, Gail said that RCTs or adaptive RCTs can be designed to address those issues in some cases, but doing so requires that the intervention and clinical question be carefully designed at the very outset of the project. He added that researchers are developing approaches to answering some of these longitudinal questions using observational data, "and to the extent that they do account for confounding by indication and for the longitudinal nature of confounding, they may be getting closer to giving good advice." Singer agreed that adaptive trial designs are a good start toward addressing longitudinal questions. Bach added that from a methodological perspective, it is "exponentially more complicated to model changes over time," referring not to the confounding issue but the mathematics.

A workshop participant from a remote site asked the panel to comment on whether it was possible to use observational studies to validate data-mining results or to use data mining as a prestep for observational studies to allow sound hypotheses to be made. Tatonetti said that data mining does in fact generate hypotheses and that the work that he presented aims to generate the best hypotheses, given the bias in the data in data sets, that can then be validated through the use of data from observational studies. He added that he was not sure that data mining had yet reached the point where it generated hypotheses better than those of an expert biologist or clinician, but that was the goal of his work.

Mary E. Charlson commented that she thought that risk prediction would benefit if the field could agree on a common set of perhaps 20 items on socioeconomic status, location, mental status, and other characteristics that everyone would collect and report in a uniform manner. Both Bach and Kattan thought this to be a great idea, but both noted that physicians may balk if the list is longer than eight items, unless the data are collected within the context of an EHR. Sheldon Greenfield remarked that he is part of a trial of elderly individuals that is trying to collect such data, and he wondered about the feasibility and cost of the use of these kinds of data to sort patients into risk groups. Bach responded that this was already being done in breast cancer prevention trials. "It is highly feasible, and in this case the effect on [the] power of selecting patients based on event probabilities is incredibly valuable," said Bach.

REFERENCES

Kattan, M. W., J. A. Eastham, A. M. Stapleton, T. M. Wheeler, and P. T. Scardino. 1998. A preoperative nomogram for disease recurrence following radical prostatectomy for prostate cancer. *Journal of the National Cancer Institute* 90(10):766–771.

Ross, P. L., C. Gerigk, M. Gonen, O. Yossepowitch, I. Cagiannos, P. C. Sogani, P. T. Scardino, and M. W. Kattan. 2002. Comparisons of nomograms and urologists' predictions in prostate cancer. *Seminars in Urologic Oncology* 20(2):82–88.

Tatonetti, N. P., J. C. Denny, S. N. Murphy, G. H. Fernald, G. Krishnan, V. Castro, P. Yue, P. S. Tsao, I. Kohane, D. M. Roden, and R. B. Altman. 2011. Detecting drug interactions from adverse-event reports: Interaction between paroxetine and pravastatin increases blood glucose levels. *Clinical Pharmacology and Therapeutics* 90(1):133–142.

Tukey, J. W. 1977. Some thoughts on clinical trials, especially problems of multiplicity. *Science* 198(4318):679–684.

Van Zee, K. J., D. M. Manasseh, J. L. Bevilacqua, S. K. Boolbol, J. V. Fey, L. K. Tan, P. I. Borgen, H. S. Cody III, and M. W. Kattan. 2003. A nomogram for predicting the likelihood of additional nodal metastases in breast cancer patients with a positive sentinel node biopsy. *Annals of Surgical Oncology* 10(10):1140–1151.

7

Strategies Going Forward

KEY SPEAKER THEMES

Mulrow

- Issues with the quality of available data sources, such as misclassification, misdiagnosis, or missing data, should be taken into account when prioritizing the funding of observational studies.
- Observational studies should be used to evaluate diagnosis, prognosis, and evaluation strategies as well as the benefits and harms of therapy.
- Clear identification of questions and outcomes of interest are important in funding observational studies and publishing their results. This can help ensure transparency and combat selective reporting.

Slutsky

- Certain study designs are appropriate for answering specific types of questions, and these questions should address the needs of decision makers.
- Few studies are robust enough to stand on their own. The field needs to start thinking in terms of a body of evidence and the quality of evidence that contributes to that body.

- Translation and dissemination of study results, and the communication and incorporation of uncertainty into decision tools are areas in need of much work in order for research to inform decision making.

Goodman

- Funding agencies such as the Patient-Centered Outcomes Research Institute (PCORI) could mandate or strongly encourage the conduct of companion randomized controlled trial (RCT) and observational studies, following patients excluded from RCTs and aligning information collection between the two methods, in order to look at the commonalities between methods and better characterize biases.
- Funding agencies, including PCORI, should fund efforts to validate different methods for exploring relationships in high-quality databases. This would be key to giving the field confidence about these methods.
- PCORI and other funders should set standards regarding the full range of expertise needed to carry out the clinical research it funds.

In the workshop's final session, three panelists aimed to capture the lessons learned over the previous day and a half of presentations and discussions. The session's three panelists—Cynthia D. Mulrow, senior deputy editor of the *Annals of Internal Medicine*; Jean R. Slutsky, director of the Center for Outcomes and Evidence, Agency for Healthcare Research and Quality (AHRQ); and Steven N. Goodman—were asked to reflect on the take-home message from the workshop and identify potential strategies to move forward.

A JOURNAL EDITOR'S PERSPECTIVE

Speaking from the perspective of an editor at a journal (the *Annals of Internal Medicine*) that publishes work that can be used to inform patient and provider decisions, Cynthia D. Mulrow said that over the previous year alone she had seen more than 1,000 papers describing observational studies but had published only about 5 percent of those papers, which she said makes her a skeptic about the value of such studies. She said that she worries that this situation is a threat to validity and to the success of the Patient-Centered Outcomes Research Institute (PCORI) and that the field may be setting overly high or overly broad expectations for many different stakeholders. She said that she worries that PCORI might "fund research that addresses nebulous questions with multiple different types of outcomes that really do not provide good information that can be used for patient decision making."

To avoid those threats, she said that PCORI needs to spend a significant amount of time identifying and prioritizing the research questions that it wants to have addressed and the research that it wants to fund and that it needs to do so with cross talk among different types of experts, whether they are clinical, patient, or methodological experts. She recommended that PCORI look at where data that measure what the field wants to have measured are available or easily collectible to ensure that the research funded not only matches a clinical question but also can supply the data needed to answer that question. Mulrow added, "I don't think we should just be amassing information for information's sake without paying any attention to things like misclassification, misdiagnosis, or large amounts of missing data that are likely to be occurring in a dataset."

Another issue that the workshop presentations raised for her was the almost exclusive focus on the benefits and harms of therapy. "Medical care focuses on things other than therapy, whether that is diagnosis or prognosis or evaluation strategies that begin a management strategy, so I would like to see PCORI spend some time and some money on funding work other than just therapy," said Mulrow.

She also said that she would have liked to have heard more about transparent reporting and selective reporting, which she believes are particular problems with observational research. She recommended that any observational studies that PCORI funds should start with clearly identified questions and outcomes of interest so that those who read the resulting papers can be assured that selective reporting has not occurred.

With respect to the last issue, Michael McGinnis asked Mulrow for suggestions on how to better capture the array of observational data or studies that are under way to improve transparency. Mulrow said that she would not recommend spending much money setting up a registry similar to clinicaltrials.gov for observational studies. "I think at this point that it behooves groups that are funding observational research to make clear that they have well-designed protocols that are available to all and that can be used throughout the process of that research," she said.

ISSUES TO CONSIDER MOVING FORWARD

Jean R. Slutsky commended the workshop presenters and participants for avoiding the observational study-versus-randomized controlled trial (RCT) conundrum and instead acknowledging the challenge inherent in combining multiple approaches to study different aspects of clinical care.

She also noted that the workshop participants paid particular attention to the fact that certain study designs are appropriate for answering specific types of questions and that these questions need to address the needs of decision makers. The latter point is often something that the field avoids discussing, she observed. She added that the important clinical questions can differ among decision makers. As an example, she cited work that AHRQ did translating the results of Mark A. Hlatky's work on percutaneous coronary intervention versus coronary artery bypass grafting to patients and clinicians. Clinicians, Slutsky said, were "obsessed with mortality as an endpoint, but patients were obsessed with angina that was disabling and got quite angry when we tried to put the dissemination document in the context of mortality."

She then listed six ideas that she gleaned from the workshop and that she thought were important for PCORI and other funding agencies such as hers, as well as for researchers. The first idea is that empirical testing is not infallible but is self-correcting. Put another way, few studies are robust enough to stand on their own. The workshop presentations were largely about individual studies and study designs, she stated, and the field needs to start thinking in terms of a body of evidence and the quality of the evidence that contributes to that body of evidence.

Slutsky's next point was that many studies are designed without rational intelligence. "Sometimes I think clinical studies are not designed with how their application will be used in decision making," she said. Next, she raised the issue that the field seldom refers to the existing body of evidence as a living, dynamic resource and instead advocates for what she referred to as "individual acronym-based studies." As a result, the field often waits on the results of some exciting clinical trial and then tries to determine how the data fit into the existing literature. Instead, the goal should be to look at the whole body of evidence and think ahead of time about the type of data that would fit with and increase the usefulness of the existing data.

The point was raised during the workshop that patients have numeracy problems, but so does the medical profession, said Slutsky, which was her fourth idea. She said that she has often been appalled at the level of misunderstanding among physicians, even those just out of medical school, about the basic constructs of relative risk versus absolute risk and progression-free survival versus mortality, for example. "We cannot assume that people understand the level at which a discussion like this takes place," she stated. "If we are not the right people to do this translation or dissemination of what this means, we have to create a body of science to make sure that happens." Along the same lines, her next idea was that the field fails to put the same emphasis on the science of how to best communicate uncertainty in the evidence for the population and the individual. Nor, she said, is the field good at incorporating uncertainty into robust tools for decision making.

For her final idea, she agreed with Mulrow that the field must demand a level of transparency in the studies that are published, particularly in how observational studies and RCTs are evaluated in systematic reviews. AHRQ, she noted, is funding the creation of a review database of studies that have been evaluated for quality, but the same level of transparency regarding inputs, algorithms, protocols, and patient-reported outcomes is needed. Transparency, she said as a final comment, is essential when one is talking about decision modeling and when one is choosing the outcomes to be measured, as those outcomes must be the ones that are important to patients.

LESSONS FROM PCORI

Steven N. Goodman, speaking from the perspective of a member of PCORI's Methodology Committee, said that the workshop provided two important lessons that can affect how the Institute acts. The first lesson, he said, pertains to the fact that PCORI is unique in being a research-funding agency with its own legislatively mandated Methodology Committee, something that, he noted, is extraordinary. The lesson is that PCORI has huge opportunities to change its review process so that it can improve the studies that it funds in a way that furthers the many goals that have been mentioned at the workshop. Instead of being a passive recipient of proposals, PCORI can play an active role in changing the culture of clinical trial design.

For example, PCORI could mandate or strongly encourage that any RCT for which a request for funding is submitted include a parallel observation study that would at a minimum follow patients who would not agree to be in the RCT but would agree to be followed. It would represent a tremendous opportunity for the field to conduct such studies in a systematic way that would provide an ongoing opportunity to develop methods for examining the factors that make RCTs and observational studies equivalent or not.

Similarly, PCORI could mandate or strongly encourage that observational studies for which a request for funding is submitted collect the same information that is gathered in related RCTs. By pushing from both sides, he said, PCORI would create opportunities to look at the commonalities between methods and characterize biases in the observational sphere. In addition, PCORI could mandate that both types of studies include more active solicitation of patient-volunteered information through the use of patient portals into the electronic health record (EHR).

The second lesson that Goodman discussed concerned the development of methods. He said that PCORI has the opportunity to fund efforts to validate different methods for exploring the relationships among data in high-quality databases. Although this type of validation work is rarely funded because it does not discover new relationships, it goes a long way, Goodman said, in giving the field confidence about the methods that it uses. He also noted the importance of development and validation of both adaptive trial designs and methods for sequential decision making in which agents are rerandomized at every key decision-making point.

As a final comment, Goodman said that the workshop clearly demonstrated the value of building a critical mass of methodologists who think deeply about the foundations of both methodology and clinical research and that he would like to see PCORI set standards for the expertise that needs to be assembled within the clinical research teams that it funds. Doing so would "institutionalize the richness of the cross talk that we saw here to make sure that the best wisdom of the best thinkers on the methodological side and on the clinical research and clinical side, as well as the patients, is brought to bear in everything that PCORI does."

DISCUSSION

Nancy Santanello said that most large pharmaceutical companies do register their observational studies on clinicaltrials.gov, though she said that doing so was difficult. She noted, too, that the European Medicines Agency now requires all observational safety studies conducted in the European Union to register with the agency using a registry that provides a more user-friendly interface for observational studies. She, and then Richard Platt, seconded the idea that everyone doing observational studies should register their studies, with Platt suggesting that funding agencies and journals require registration as a requirement for funding or publication. Slutsky added that the American Recovery and Reinvestment Act of 2009 funded a patient registry to be integrated into clinicaltrials.gov, though linking of observational studies to the registry is voluntary.

Platt then commented that, in his view, the value of claims data combined with the ability to conduct a full review of the text records for selected patients is underappreciated. An advantage to the use of claims data, he said, is that the population is well-defined and coverage is reasonably complete over the defined time period. At the same time, he believed that the field may be overestimating the ease with which EHR data can be used. In a final remark, Platt suggested that the National Institutes of Health Collaboratory would be a good partner for PCORI if PCORI wants to follow the recommendations to take a more active role in trial design.

Sean Hennessy said that although data-mining approaches have good sensitivity when it comes to identifying adverse drug events, the real issue is specificity, and thus, good methods for evaluating specificity are needed. Following up on Slutsky's observation that the results of one study are rarely a sufficient basis to change clinical practice widely, he said that both AHRQ and PCORI are asking researchers to disseminate their findings into practice as soon as they have them. He voiced concern that PCORI could run into trouble over the implementation of results that should not be implemented yet. Slutsky replied that AHRQ has always emphasized considering the audience for dissemination. With the results of a single study, unless they are remarkably definitive, the audience should be other researchers and funding agencies and not the general public.

Joe V. Selby added that PCORI does not ask its applicants to even plan for dissemination. What PCORI does do is ask its applicants to assess the potential for dissemination and to outline what the applicants perceive to be opportunities, should the findings warrant dissemination. He noted that PCORI is working with AHRQ to develop a broad-based dissemination plan. Mulrow remarked that consideration should also be given to how evidence from observational studies should be synthesized before being disseminated.

Sheldon Greenfield asked if it would be possible to create a family of studies with the goal of having the combined findings of these studies in, say, 4 years provide clinical practice guideline makers and systematic reviewers with enough of the right kind of data to make some kind of statement. Goodman added that although it is important to keep a balance between allowing individual investigators to develop their own ideas and to have central control, it should be possible for PCORI to bring together investigators who work in the same field to standardize measures in their studies and perhaps provide an overview that would enable meta-analysis at the end of the studies. "PCORI, as well as NIH [National Institutes of Health], can take the initiative by convening conferences to help standardize these measures across bodies of research," Goodman said in support of Greenfield's suggestion. "I think PCORI and other funding agencies can do it without being too dictatorial and start establishing the infrastructure, both intellectual and substantive, for research in high-priority areas to go forward efficiently."

Miguel A. Hernán commented on the importance of data quality and selective reporting of multiple comparisons. He said that these are at least as important as confounding, and he encouraged funding agencies to pay attention to research on the importance of biases due to both poor data quality and selective reporting on multiple comparisons. He disagreed with the idea of registering observational studies because of the challenge of selective reporting of multiple comparisons and said that methods for quantifying the magnitude of the problem of selective reporting are needed. Santanello argued that registration is important because it forces investigators to write a protocol, ask a scientific question, and develop a plan to analyze the data.

Making the session's final comment, Patrick Ryan noted that although data quality is important, the key point that Mulrow raised is that the analysis of the data being performed must be valid. "If job number one is generating the highest-quality evidence possible," he said, "we need to figure out a framework for how to evaluate how much we can believe the result that is generated when a particular method is applied to a particular data source."

CLOSING REMARKS

In his closing remarks, Ralph I. Horwitz said that one conclusion that he drew from the workshop is that it is not enough to document when conflicts exist among randomized trials and among observational studies or between them, nor is it enough to document when conflicts exist around treatment heterogeneity. In his opinion, observational research would be advanced enormously if more attention was paid to understanding the sources of conflict in results both within observational studies and between observational studies and randomized trials. Understanding why studies give differing results will be key to helping improve them.

He also said that he hoped that the workshop would help expand the scope of information that contributes to both observational research and RCTs and that investigators would pay more attention to collecting data on the patient experience and using those data to better inform decision making to benefit the patient.

In his closing remarks, Selby summarized some of what he learned from written comments that workshop participants submitted during the lunch break. Many of the comments called for more complete data, higher-quality data, more observations, and more data per observation. They also highlighted the need for more granular data and different types of data, particularly data from the patient's perspective. He acknowledged the suggestion that PCORI fund empirical studies on the impact of differences in the quality of data and on validation of the results of studies found in one setting with those of studies found in other settings.

Other comments noted the importance of the conduct of simple, clustered RCTs and of consideration of informed consent at both the patient and the institutional levels. The role of biology in disease and biomarkers in treatment effectiveness was raised, as was the role of socioeconomic status.

As a final comment, Selby addressed the subject of the learning health care system and said, "there is not any doubt that if we want research that reflects real-world practice and if we want research that changes real-world practice, the research is going to have to be done in that real world." That real world is composed of many types of health care systems, and it is going to take the active consent of those systems to host the activities that will make high-quality research a reality. It will be up to the field to demonstrate to those health care systems the benefit of participating in research. That will require careful thinking about the needs of those systems in formulating the questions that trials will be designed to answer.

8

Common Themes for Progress

THEMES

Methods

- Greater rigor is needed in the use of observational methods; even the best methods used incorrectly will yield bad results. (Goodman)
- No one method is infallible, multiple methods are needed to answer a question and inform decision making. (Slutsky)
- Validating methods for exploring relationships in high-quality databases is critical to understanding how large databases might best contribute to evidence generation. (Ryan)
- The right question must be asked, and the right analytic methods applied, in order to validly compare observational studies and randomized controlled trials (RCTs). (Hernán and Kaizar)
- A better understanding is needed of the fundamental biologic differences that drive treatment effect heterogeneity. (Horwitz)

Policy

- Funder requirements for parallel observational studies and RCTs assessing the same question can aid in evaluating the validity and generalizing results of both approaches. (Goodman)

- Registration of observational studies in databases such as clinicaltrials.gov may counteract the selective reporting of studies and eliminate needless repetition of studies. (Santanello)
- Greater transparency in the publication of approaches and methods used, particularly in how observational studies and RCTs are evaluated in systematic reviews, can help the interpretation of results to inform decision making. (Mulrow and Slutsky)

Stakeholder Engagement

- Stakeholder engagement is critical in order for studies to be maximally useful to decision makers, and stakeholder engagement of patients and providers is critical. Studies should be pegged to their interests and evidence needs and be paired with the most appropriate methods to deliver actionable results. (Slutsky)
- Challenges such as innumeracy and a lack of understanding of uncertainty will require consideration when approaching the use and dissemination of observational studies results. (Slutsky)

A number of common themes emerged from the workshop presentations and discussions. These themes both touched on the role of observational studies as contributors to clinical evidence and identified priorities for innovation in the methods of conduct of clinical trials on the basis of current gaps and shortfalls. Participants and speakers shared their thoughts on changes in policies, particularly those of funders and journal editors, that can move research toward producing practical evidence useful to health care decision making. Finally, the engagement of stakeholders, patients, clinicians, researchers, and health systems was a common subject of discussion.

METHODS

Workshop participants who spoke and speakers cautioned against over-simplification of the discussion on the use of appropriate methods to inform decision making. Steven N. Goodman called for greater rigor in the use of observational methods, reminding everyone that even the best methods used incorrectly will yield bad results. The need for the use of multiple methods to answer a question was highlighted, and it was noted that few studies are robust enough to stand on their own and that no one method is infallible.

To get a better understanding of how large databases might best contribute to the generation of evidence, the validation of methods for exploring relationships in high-quality databases was highlighted. Patrick Ryan suggested that the creation of a reference set of positive and negative controls in the context of comparative effectiveness research, as the Observational Medical Outcomes Partnership has done for safety, would be one approach to aid the validation effort. At the same time, validation of novel approaches to experimental methodologies, such as adaptive trial designs and methods, to bolster both observational and experimental approaches was mentioned. The specific development of observational analogs of intent-to-treat and per-protocol-effect methods to allow broader application of innovative statistical methods was highlighted.

In making comparisons between observational studies and randomized controlled trials (RCTs), Miguel A. Hernán and Eloise E. Kaizar emphasized the importance of ensuring that the questions asked be the same and that the confounders be well understood so that comparisons are of apples to apples. Better understanding of the quality of the data available from observational studies, the implications of the quality of the data for use of the evidence, and approaches to improve those data and mitigate current problems were all suggested to be crucial to ensuring that the use of innovative methods leads to the production of credible, useable evidence. The increased capture and use of patient-centered outcomes and patient-contributed data were suggested to be priorities in this area.

Several workshop participants called for the need to move beyond discussions of whether treatment effect heterogeneity is real to better understanding of the fundamental biologic differences which are likely the main source of heterogeneity. Kent highlighted the limitations of current approaches, including analytical approaches that cannot contend with studies that are under-powered to detect sub-group effects and the one-variable-at-a-time approach to subgroup analysis. Instead approaches assessing combinations of variables were suggested, such as multivariate risk models.

POLICY

Workshop presentations and discussions reinforced the importance of observational studies as a component of a robust clinical research enterprise. They emphasized their complementarity to other methods in supporting health care decision making and highlighted the importance that they receive continued support from funders and be considered to provide valuable contributions by tenure and promotion committees. Encouragement of greater collection and use of patient-contributed information in observational research was also noted to be a priority for funder engagement.

Several participants made specific suggestions on how the complemen tarity of observational studies and RCTs could be improved, including the suggestion that observational studies with patients excluded from an RCT be run in parallel. Participants who spoke suggested that this could be done through the use of mechanisms such as registries and could be encouraged by funder and journal requirements. In addition, Steven N. Goodman pointed out, this would be a tremendous opportunity for the development of methods for examining factors that make RCTs and observational studies equivalent or not.

Jean R. Slutsky noted that the field of clinical research needs to start thinking in terms of a body of evidence and the quality of the evidence that contributes to that body of evidence. One of the challenges to this perspective that participants cited is the lack of transparency in observational study methods and the reporting of their results. Selective reporting is a major hindrance to being able to consider the full body of evidence around a research question and can lead to unnecessary repetition of studies and wasted resources. Registration of observational studies, either as part of the clinicaltrial.gov database or through the creation of a new database, was suggested to be one way to mitigate this issue.

In thinking about the dissemination of research results to inform decision making, Slutsky called for greater transparency in published studies, particularly in how observational studies and RCTs are evaluated in systematic reviews. The development of a framework to organize the evidence and evaluate when the evidence is good enough to inform decision making, depending on the methods used and the data source, was suggested to be a practical approach to address this.

STAKEHOLDER ENGAGEMENT

Greater stakeholder engagement around observational studies and their role in supporting health care decisions was a theme of many of the discussions throughout the workshop.

Participants who spoke repeatedly noted that for studies to be maximally useful to stakeholders, they must be pegged to stakeholder interests and evidence needs and be paired with methods that are the most appropriate to the delivery of actionable results. Stakeholder engagement, particularly patients, clinicians, and health care delivery systems, in research priority setting was cited as an important step in realizing this goal. Engagement of clinicians as the collectors of data and the consumers of the evidence generated by clinical research was highlighted as being critical to the ability to carry out high-quality studies and to ensure that study findings have an impact on clinical practice. Similarly, in order to dedicate staff time and resources to observational studies, they should be valuable to health care delivery systems. Several speaker and workshop participants who spoke suggested that patients, the ultimate stakeholders in health care decisions, should be at the center of the research questions for the results to be maximally useful in informing their decisions and in building a foundation for their participation in clinical research.

Workshop participants who spoke highlighted several challenges to a broader approach to stakeholder engagement. The issue of innumeracy, or a lack of familiarity with mathematical concepts, was highlighted as a challenge of particular import for both patients and clinicians.

With this issue in mind, the use of targeted communication strategies was suggested to be an approach to more effective communication about the value of observational studies and to the dissemination of results. Several workshop participants who spoke highlighted similar issues around challenges communicating uncertainty to individual patients, clinicians, and the population. In addition to the use of targeted communication strategies, the incorporation of uncertainty into robust tools for decision making was suggested.

Appendix A

Biographies of Workshop Speakers

Peter Bach, MD, MAPP, holds research interests in health care policy, particularly as it relates to Medicare, racial disparities in cancer care quality, and the epidemiology of lung cancer. His research examining quality of care for Medicare beneficiaries has demonstrated that blacks do not receive care that is of as high a quality as that received by whites when they are diagnosed with lung cancer and that the aptitude and resources of primary care physicians who treat blacks are inferior to those of primary care physicians who primarily treat whites. In 2007, he was the senior author of a study demonstrating that care in Medicare is highly fragmented, with the average beneficiary seeing multiple primary care physicians and specialists. His work in lung cancer epidemiology has focused on the development and utilization of lung cancer prediction models that can be used to determine what lung cancer events that populations of elderly smokers will experience over a period of time. His health care policy analysis includes investigations into Medicare's approaches to cancer payment, as well as the development of models of alternative reimbursement, payment systems, and coverage policies. He is funded by grants from the National Institute of Aging, a contract from the National Cancer Institute, and philanthropic sources. He formerly served as a senior adviser to the administrator of the Centers for Medicare & Medicaid Services (CMS). He serves on several national committees, including the Institute of Medicine's National Cancer Policy Forum and the Committee on Performance Measurement of the National Committee on Quality Assurance. He chairs the Technical Expert Panel that is developing measures of cancer care quality for CMS. Along with publishing in medical literature, Bach's opinion pieces have appeared in numerous lay news outlets, including the *New York Times*, the *Wall Street Journal*, *Forbes Online*, and National Public Radio.

Anirban Basu, PhD, is an associate professor in the departments of health services, pharmacy, and economics at the University of Washington, Seattle, and directs the Program in Health Economics and Outcomes Methodology there. He is also a faculty research fellow at the National Bureau of Economic Research. Dr. Basu received his MS in biostatistics from the University of North Carolina at Chapel Hill in 1999 and his PhD in public policy from the University of Chicago in 2004. Dr. Basu works at the interface of microeconomics, statistics, and health policy. His work has enriched the theoretical foundations of comparative and cost-effectiveness analyses. He has developed innovative methods to study heterogeneity in clinical and economic outcomes in order to establish the value of individualized care. His works have appeared in many leading peer-reviewed journals, including *Journal of Health Economics*, *Health Economics*, *PharmacoEconomics*, *Statistics in Medicine*, *Biostatistics*, *Medical Decision Making*, and others. Dr. Basu is an associate editor for both *Health Economics* and the *Journal of Health Economics* and has taught courses on health economics, decision analysis, cost-effectiveness analysis, and health services research methods. He has received numerous recognitions for his work throughout his career: the NARSAD Wodecroft Young Investigator Award (2005), the Research Excellence Award for Methodological Excellence (2007), and the Bernie O'Brien New Investigator Award (2009) from the International Society for Pharmacoeconomics and Outcomes Research, the Alan Williams Health Economics Fellowship (2008) from the University of York, United Kingdom, and the Labelle Lectureship in Health Economics (2009) from McMaster University, Canada.

Robert M. Califf, MD, Vice Chancellor for Clinical and Translational Research, director of the Duke Translational Medicine Institute (DTMI), and professor of medicine in the Division of Cardiology at Duke University Medical Center in Durham, North Carolina, leads a multifaceted organization that seeks to transform how scientific discoveries are translated into improved health outcomes. Before leading DTMI, he was the founding director of the Duke Clinical Research Institute, one of the nation's premier academic research organizations. He is editor in chief of the *American Heart Journal*, the oldest cardiovascular specialty journal, and a practicing cardiologist at Duke University Medical Center.

Mary E. Charlson, MD, is the William T. Foley Distinguished Professor in Medicine, the executive director of the Center for Integrative Medicine and the chief of the Division of Clinical Epidemiology and Evaluative Sciences Research at Weill Medical College of Cornell University/New York Presbyterian Hospital. She is also the program chairperson for the master of science program in clinical epidemiology and health services research and director of the Agency for Healthcare Research and Quality. Dr. Charlson is an international leader in the measurement and improvement of risk-adjusted outcomes and developed a method of assessing the prognostic impact of comorbid conditions; the Charlson Comorbidity Index, which is one of the most widely utilized measurements in chronic disease. She is the principal investigator of the National Heart, Lung, and Blood Institute Small Changes and Lasting Effects, a randomized trial aimed to reduce weight among overweight/obese Black and Latino adults living primarily in Harlem and the South Bronx, through small changes in eating behavior and physical activity. She is co–principal investigator of the National Institute on Minority Health and Health Disparities' Center for Excellence in Health Disparities Research and Community Engagement, which conducts health disparities research. Dr. Charlson received her MD from Yale University School of Medicine. After completing her residency at Johns Hopkins Hospital, she was a Robert Wood Johnson Clinical Scholar at Yale.

Mark R. Cullen, MD, is professor of medicine and chief of the Division of General Medical Disciplines at Stanford University. Trained in internal medicine and occupational health, he has devoted his research career to the study of the role of work, including social, physical, and economic dimensions, in the evolution of chronic disease, disability, and death. The focus of early work was the impact of physical and chemical hazards, including metals, solvents, and mineral dusts. In 1997, he was invited to join the Macarthur Foundation Research Network on Socioeconomic Status and Health. During the same year he entered into a long-term research agreement with Alcoa, a multinational aluminum producer, to study the determinants of health in Alcoa's large stable workforce, for which exceptionally rich environmental, social, economic, and medical data were available; this has formed the basis of the multidisciplinary Alcoa study, which now includes researchers and trainees in medical and social sciences at a dozen academic institutions and which is primarily supported by funds from the National Institutes of Health. To date, the study has generated some 40 publications and about a dozen doctoral theses. In addition to this long-standing project, Dr. Cullen has embarked on the study of determinants of differences in premature mortality by race, sex, and geography both in U.S. counties and globally. Another new area of research involves development of methods to assess the impact of social and physical environments in large population studies to better understand how these factors, along with genetics, contribute to the risk for the development of chronic disease. Dr. Cullen is a faculty research fellow of the National Bureau of Economic Research and was elected to the Institute of Medicine of the National Academy of Sciences in 1997.

Mitchell H. Gail, MD, PhD, is a senior investigator in the Biostatistics Branch of the Division of Cancer Epidemiology and Genetics, National Cancer Institute. He received an MD from Harvard Medical School and a PhD in statistics from George Washington University. His work at the National Cancer Institute included studies on the motility of cells in tissue culture; clinical trials of lung cancer treatments and preventive interventions for gastric cancer; and assessment of cancer biomarkers, AIDS epidemiology, and models to project the risk of breast cancer. Dr. Gail's current research interests include statistical methods for the design and analysis of epidemiological studies, including studies of genetic factors, and models to predict the absolute risk of disease. Dr. Gail is a fellow and former president of the American Statistical Association and a member of the Institute of Medicine of the National Academy of Sciences.

Steven N. Goodman, MD, MHS, PhD, is associate dean for clinical and translational research and professor of medicine and health policy and research at the Stanford University School of Medicine. Before joining Stanford in 2011, Dr. Goodman was professor of oncology in the division of biostatistics of the Johns Hopkins Kimmel Cancer Center, with appointments in the departments of pediatrics, biostatistics, and epidemiology in the Johns Hopkins Schools of Medicine and Public Health. At Johns Hopkins he was co-director of the epidemiology doctoral program for 7 years and led two major curriculum design efforts. He is the editor of *Clinical Trials: Journal of the Society for Clinical Trials* and senior statistical editor for the *Annals of Internal Medicine*, where he has been since 1987. He has served on a wide range of Institute of Medicine committees, including Agent Orange and Veterans, Immunization Safety, Treatment of PTSD in Veterans, and most recently co-chaired the Committee on Ethical and Scientific Issues in Studying the Safety of Approved Drugs. Dr. Goodman served on the Surgeon General's committee to write the 2004 report on the Health Consequences of Smoking. He is a scientific advisor to the Medical Advisory Panel of the National Blue Cross/Blue Shield Technology Evaluation Center, and in 2011 was appointed by the Government Accountability Office to the Methodology Committee of the Patient-Centered Outcomes Research Institute. Dr. Goodman received a BA from Harvard, an MD from New York University, trained in pediatrics at Washington University in St. Louis, obtaining board certification, and received an MHS in biostatistics and PhD in epidemiology from Johns Hopkins University. He writes and teaches on evidence evaluation and inferential, methodological, and ethical issues in clinical research, epidemiology, and comparative effectiveness research.

Joel B. Greenhouse, PhD, is professor of statistics at Carnegie Mellon University and adjunct professor of psychiatry and epidemiology at the University of Pittsburgh. He is a fellow of the American Statistical Association and of the American Association for the Advancement of Science and an elected member of the International Statistical Institute. Dr. Greenhouse has been a member of the National Academy of Sciences' Committee on National Statistics, the Institute of Medicine's Committee on the Assessment of Family Violence Interventions, and the National Research Council's Panel on Statistical Issues for Research in the Combination of Information. He is an editor of the journal *Statistics in Medicine* and is a past editor of the Institute of Mathematical Statistics' *Lecture Notes and Monograph Series*. His research interests include methods for the analysis of data from longitudinal and observational studies and methods for clinical trials. Dr. Greenhouse is also interested in issues related to the use of research synthesis in practice, especially as it is used to synthesize evidence for scientific discovery and for making policy.

Miguel A. Hernán, MD, DrPH, is a professor for the departments of epidemiology and biostatistics, Harvard School of Public Health, and an affiliated faculty member of the Harvard–Massachusetts Institute of Technology Division of Health Sciences and Technology. He is the editor of *Epidemiology*, associate editor of the *Journal of the American Statistical Association* and the *American Journal of Epidemiology*, principal investigator of the HIVCAUSAL Collaboration (a consortium of prospective studies of human immunodeficiency virus [HIV]-infected individuals from Europe and the United States), and a fellow of the American Association for the Advancement of Science. He writes and teaches on methodology for causal inference, including comparative effectiveness of policy and clinical interventions. His applied research interests include the optimal use of antiretroviral therapy for HIV disease, clinical strategies to reduce mortality after kidney failure, and lifestyle and pharmacologic interventions to reduce the incidence of cardiovascular disease. He served on the Institute of Medicine's Committee on Ethical and Scientific Issues in Studying the Safety of Approved Drugs and currently serves on the National Research Council's Committee to Review the IRIS Process.

Mark A. Hlatky, MD, is professor of health research and policy and professor of medicine (cardiovascular medicine) at Stanford University. He is a cardiologist with major research interests in clinical research methods, outcomes research, and clinical trials. Dr. Hlatky has participated in several large, multicenter randomized clinical trials, including studies of coronary revascularization, treatment of acute myocardial infarction, hormone therapy to prevent cardiovascular disease, and management of life-threatening ventricular arrhythmias. He has also conducted large outcomes research studies of the comparative effectiveness of coronary revascularization procedures and of drug treatments for heart disease. He is currently studying methods for assessing how the effectiveness of treatments is modified by patient characteristics and how to apply these methods to personalize treatment recommendations. Dr. Hlatky has served on numerous national advisory panels and clinical guideline committees and is the associate editor of the *Journal of the American College of Cardiology*.

Ralph I. Horwitz, MD, MACP, is senior vice president for clinical evaluation sciences and senior advisor to the chairman of research and development at GlaxoSmithKline (GSK), and Harold H. Hines, Jr. Professor Emeritus of medicine and epidemiology at Yale University. Dr. Horwitz trained in internal medicine at institutions (Royal Victoria Hospital of McGill University and the Massachusetts General Hospital) where science and clinical medicine were connected effortlessly. These experiences as a resident unleashed a deep interest in clinical research training that he pursued as a fellow in the Robert Wood Johnson Clinical Scholars Program at Yale under the direction of Alvan R. Feinstein. He joined the Yale faculty in 1978 and remained there for 25 years as co-director of the Clinical Scholars Program and later as chair of the department of medicine. Before joining GSK, Dr. Horwitz was chair of medicine at Stanford University and dean of Case Western Reserve Medical School. He is an elected member of the Institute of Medicine of the National Academy of Sciences; the American Society for Clinical Investigation; the American Epidemiological Society; and the Association of American Physicians (he was president in 2010). He was a member of the advisory committee to the National Institutes of Health director (under both Elias Zerhouni and Francis Collins). Dr. Horwitz served on the American Board of Internal Medicine and was chairman in 2003. He is a master of the American College of Physicians.

Eloise E. Kaizar, PhD, is associate professor of statistics at The Ohio State University. She received a doctorate in statistics from Carnegie Mellon University in 2006. Her primary research focus is on assessing the efficacy and safety of medical interventions, especially those whose effects are heterogeneous across populations or that are measured with rare event outcomes. As such, she has worked on a methodology to combine multiple sources of information relevant to, but perhaps containing different kinds of information about, the same broad policy or patient-centered question. She is particularly interested in how data collected via different study designs (randomized trials, administrative data, or sample surveys) can contribute complementary information. Dr. Kaizar also examines statistical methodology to identify and verify subpopulations for whom treatment is particularly effective and safe. Her work has appeared in a variety of journals, including *Statistics in Medicine* and the *Journal of the American Statistical Association.*

Michael W. Kattan, MBA, PhD, is chairman of the Department of Quantitative Health Sciences at The Cleveland Clinic and professor of medicine, epidemiology, and biostatistics at the Cleveland Clinic Lerner College of Medicine of Case Western Reserve University. Dr. Kattan has a PhD in management information systems with a minor in statistics. He also holds an MBA with a concentration in quantitative sciences. Following his studies, he completed a postdoctoral program in medical informatics before joining the faculty at the Baylor College of Medicine in Houston, Texas. He has published more than 350 peer-reviewed publications and is best known for his prediction models, called nomograms, in various cancers. He has received two patents for this work and serves on the editorial boards for *Cancer Investigation* and *Nature Clinical Practice Urology.* Dr. Kattan is interested in the development, validation, and use of prediction models. He has developed several such models in cancer and released them as freely available software from www.nomograms.org. Dr. Kattan is also interested in quality-of-life assessment to support medical decision making, such as utility assessment. Other interests include decision analysis and cost-effectiveness analysis.

David M. Kent, MD, MSc, is director of the clinical and translational science (CTS) MS/PhD program at the Sackler School of Graduate Biomedical Sciences at Tufts University and associate professor of medicine, neurology, and CTS at the Tufts Medical Center/Tufts University School of Medicine. A general internist, Dr. Kent is a clinician-methodologist most interested in the problems of making inferences to individual patients based on effects measured in groups. He has a broad background in clinical epidemiology with a focus on predictive modeling in cardiovascular and cerebrovascular disease, as well as experience in meta-analytic approaches, particularly individual patient data (IPD) meta-analysis. Dr. Kent has substantial experience leading collaborative projects involving the secondary analysis of large clinical trial databases. Prior federally funded work involving IPD meta-analysis includes predictive modeling to balance patient-specific risks and benefits for thrombolytics in acute stroke, a project that pooled data from 6 clinical trials, and for coronary reperfusion therapy, which combined 10 databases. Dr. Kent is also the principal investigator (PI) of the National Institute of Neurological Disorders and Stroke–sponsored Risk of Paradoxical Embolism Study, pooling 12 observational databases to create predictive models to be applied to 3 on-going clinical trials. His research also addresses fundamental analytic issues in how to employ a risk-modeling approach to clinical trial analysis, and he is currently the PI of a Patient-Centered Outcomes Research Institute–funded methods project in this area.

Michael Lauer, MD, is the director of the Division of Cardiovascular Sciences at the National Heart, Lung, and Blood Institute (NHLBI), part of the National Institutes of Health. In this position, Dr. Lauer provides leadership for the institute's national program for research on the causes, prevention, and treatment of cardiovascular (basic, clinical, population, and health sciences) diseases. Dr. Lauer joined NHLBI in July 2007. Dr. Lauer's primary research interests include cardiovascular clinical epidemiology and comparative effectiveness, with a focus on diagnostic testing. He also has a strong background in leadership of the cardiovascular community and longstanding interests in medical editing—for 7 years he was a contributing editor for the *Journal of the American Medical Association*—and human subjects protection. Prior to joining NHLBI, Dr. Lauer served as the director of the Cleveland Clinic Foundation Exercise Laboratory and vice chair of the clinic's institutional review board. He also served as co-director of the Coronary Intensive Care Unit and director of clinical research in the clinic's department of cardiology. Dr. Lauer earned his BS in biology, summa cum laude, from Rensselaer Polytechnic Institute in 1983 and his MD, magna cum laude, from Albany Medical College in 1985. Following internal medical training at the Massachusetts General Hospital, Harvard Medical School, he completed a clinical fellowship in cardiology at the Boston Beth Israel Hospital, Harvard Medical School. His further training in epidemiology included a research fellowship at the NHLBI's Framingham Heart Study, Boston University; the program in clinical effectiveness, Harvard School of Public Health, Harvard University; and the Program for Physician Educators, Harvard Macy Institute. Dr. Lauer is an elected fellow of the American College of Cardiology and American Heart Association (AHA), and has been elected to membership in the American Society for Clinical Investigation. He also served as chairman of the Exercise, Cardiac Rehabilitation, and Prevention Committee of AHA's Council of Clinical Cardiology, and has received numerous awards in recognition of his scientific and teaching accomplishments.

J. Michael McGinnis, MD, MPP, is a physician, epidemiologist, and longtime contributor to national and international health programs and policy. An elected member of the Institute of Medicine (IOM) of the National Academy of Sciences, he has since 2005 also served as IOM senior scholar and executive director of the IOM Roundtable on Value & Science-Driven

Health Care. He founded and stewards the IOM's Learning Health System initiative and, in prior posts, also served as founding leader for the Robert Wood Johnson Foundation's (RWJF's) Health Group, the World Bank/ European Commission Task Force for Health Reconstruction in Bosnia, and, in the U.S. government, the Office of Research Integrity, the Nutrition Policy Board, and the Office of Disease Prevention and Health Promotion. In the last post, he held continuous policy responsibilities for prevention through four administrations (those of Presidents Jimmy Carter, Ronald Reagan, George H. W. Bush, and Bill Clinton), during which he conceived and launched a number of initiatives of ongoing policy importance, including the Healthy People national goals and objectives, the U.S. Preventive Services Task Force, the Dietary Guidelines for Americans, and development of the Ten Essential Services of Public Health. At RWJF, he founded the Health & Society Scholars program, the Young Epidemiology Scholars program, and the Active Living family of programs. Early in his career he served in India as an epidemiologist and state director for the World Health Organization's Smallpox Eradication Program. Widely published, he has made foundational contributions to understanding the basic determinants of health (e.g., "Actual Causes of Death," *Journal of the American Medical Association* 270:18, 1993, and "The Case for More Active Policy Attention to Health Promotion," *Health Affairs* 21:2, 2002). National leadership awards include the Arthur S. Flemming Award, the Distinguished Service Award for public health leadership, the Health Leader of the Year Award, and the Public Health Hero Award. He has held visiting or adjunct professorships at George Washington University, the University of California, Los Angeles (UCLA), Princeton University, and Duke University. He is a graduate of the University of California, Berkeley, the UCLA School of Medicine, and the John F. Kennedy School of Government at Harvard University and was the graduating commencement speaker at each.

Sally C. Morton, PhD, is professor and chair of biostatistics and director of the Comparative Effectiveness Research Core at the University of Pittsburgh. Previously, she was vice president for statistics and epidemiology at RTI International and head of the RAND Corporation Statistics Group. Her research interests include the use of statistics in evidence-based medicine, particularly meta-analysis. She serves as a statistical expert for the Patient-Centered Outcomes Research Institute Methodology Committee and as an evidence synthesis expert for Agency for Healthcare Research and Quality Evidence-Based Practice Centers. She has been a member of several Institute of Medicine committees on comparative effectiveness research, geographic variations in Medicare and systematic reviews, and serves on the National Academy of Sciences' Committee on National Statistics. She received a PhD in statistics from Stanford University.

Cynthia D. Mulrow, MD, MSc, MACP, is senior deputy editor of the *Annals of Internal Medicine* and clinical professor of medicine at the University of Texas Health Science Center at San Antonio. She has been a program director of the Robert Wood Johnson Foundation Generalist Physician Faculty Scholars Program and director of the San Antonio Cochrane Collaboration Center and the San Antonio Evidence-Based Practice Center. She was elected to the American Society of Clinical Investigation in 1997, honored as a master of the American College of Physicians in 2005, and elected to the Institute of Medicine in 2008. Dr. Mulrow's academic work followed several themes, including systematic reviews, evidence synthesis, practice guidelines, research methodology, and chronic medical conditions. Early in her career, she published the article "The Medical Review Article: State of the Science" (*Annals of Internal Medicine* 106:485–488, 1987). She followed it with publication of a series of articles in the *Annals of Internal Medicine* and a book, *Systematic Reviews and Synthesis of Best Evidence for Health Care Decisions*. She also authored several information syntheses and technology reports and served on several guideline panels, including the U.S. Preventive Services Task Force. She currently contributes to three groups that set standards for reporting research: PRISMA (systematic reviews and meta-analyses), STROBE (observational studies), and CONSORT (clinical trials).

Richard Platt, MD, MS, is professor and chair of the Harvard Medical School department of population medicine at the Harvard Pilgrim Health Care Institute, Boston, Massachusetts. He is the principal investigator of the Food and Drug Administration Mini-Sentinel program, of a Centers for Disease Control and Prevention (CDC) Prevention Epicenter, a CDC Center of Excellence in Public Health Informatics, and an Agency for Healthcare Research and Quality DEcIDE center. He is a member of the Institute of Medicine Roundtable on Value & Science-Driven Health Care and co-chair of its Clinical Effectiveness Research Innovation Collaborative. He is also a member of the American Association of Medical Colleges Advisory Panel on Research.

Patrick Ryan, PhD, is the head of epidemiology analytics at Johnson & Johnson Pharmaceutical Research and Development, where he has leading efforts to develop and apply analysis methods to better understand the effects of medical products. He also currently serves as a research investigator of the Observational Medical Outcomes Partnership, a public–private partnership chaired by the Food and Drug Administration. As part of this effort, he is conducting methodological research to assess the appropriate use of observational health care data to identify and evaluate drug safety issues.

Sebastian Schneeweiss, MD, ScD, is professor of medicine and epidemiology at Harvard Medical School and vice chief of the Division of Pharmacoepidemiology and Pharmacoeconomics of the Department of Medicine, Brigham and Women's Hospital (BWH). He is principal investigator of the BWH DEcIDE Research Center on Comparative Effectiveness Research and the DEcIDE Methods Center, both funded by Agency for Healthcare Research and Quality, and director of the Harvard-Brigham Drug Safety Research Center, funded by the Center for Drug Evaluation and Research, U.S. Food and Drug Administration (FDA). His research is funded by multiple National Institutes of Health grants and focuses on the comparative effectiveness and safety of biopharmaceuticals and analytic methods to improve the validity of epidemiological studies through the use of complex health care databases, particularly for newly marketed medical products. His work is published in high-ranking journals and was featured in *Discover* magazine. Dr. Schneeweiss is past president of the International Society for Pharmacoepidemiology and is a fellow of the American College of Epidemiology, the American College of Clinical Pharmacology, and the International Society for Pharmacoepidemiology. He is a voting consultant to the FDA Drug Safety and Risk Management Advisory Committee and a member of the Methods Committee of the Patient-Centered Outcomes Research Institute. He received his medical training at the University of Munich Medical School and a doctoral degree in pharmacoepidemiology from Harvard University.

Joe V. Selby, MD, MPH, is the first executive director of the Patient-Centered Outcomes Research Institute (PCORI). A family physician, clinical epidemiologist, and health services researcher, he has more than 35 years of experience in patient care, research, and administration. He will identify strategic issues and opportunities for PCORI and implement and administer programs authorized by the PCORI Board of Governors. Building on the work of the board and interim staff, Dr. Selby will lead the organizational development of PCORI, which was established by Congress through the 2010 Patient Protection and Affordable Care Act. In addition to creating an organizational structure to carry out a national research agenda, Dr. Selby will lead PCORI's external communications, including work to establish effective two-way communication channels with the public and stakeholders about PCORI's work. Dr. Selby joined PCORI from Kaiser Permanente, Northern California, where he was director of the division of research for 13 years and oversaw a department of more than 50 investigators and 500 research staff working on more than 250 ongoing studies. He was with Kaiser Permanente for 27 years. An accomplished researcher, Dr. Selby has authored more than 200 peer-reviewed articles and continues to conduct research, primarily in the areas of diabetes outcomes and quality improvement. His publications cover a spectrum of topics, including effectiveness studies of colorectal cancer screening strategies; treatment effectiveness, population management, and disparities in diabetes mellitus; and primary care delivery and quality measurement. Dr. Selby was elected to membership in the Institute of Medicine in 2009 and was a member of the Agency for Healthcare Research and Quality study section for Health Care Quality and Effectiveness from 1999 to 2003. A native of Fulton, Missouri, Dr. Selby received his medical degree from Northwestern University and his master's in public health from the University of California, Berkeley. He was a commissioned officer in the Public Health Service from 1976 to 1983 and received the Commissioned Officer's Award in 1981. He serves as lecturer in the department of epidemiology and biostatistics at the University of California, San Francisco, School of Medicine, and as a consulting professor, health research and policy at the Stanford University School of Medicine.

Burton Singer, PhD, MS, is adjunct professor in the Emerging Pathogens Institute and department of mathematics at the University of Florida. From 1993 to July 2009, he was the Charles & Marie Robertson Professor of Public and International Affairs at Princeton University. He has served as chair of the National Research Council's Committee on National Statistics and as chair of the Steering Committee for Social and Economic Research in the World Health Organization Tropical Disease Research program. He has centered his research in three principal areas: identification of social, biological, and environmental risks associated with vector-borne diseases in the tropics; integration of psychosocial and biological evidence to characterize pathways to alternative states of health; and health impact assessments associated with economic development projects. He was elected to the National Academy of Sciences (1994) and the Institute of Medicine of the National Academy of Sciences (2005) and was a Guggenheim Fellow in 1981–1982. He received his PhD in statistics from Stanford University in 1967.

Jean R. Slutsky, PA, MS, has directed the Center for Outcomes and Evidence (COE), Agency for Healthcare Research and Quality (AHRQ) of the U.S. Department of Health and Human Services since June 2003. Prior to Ms. Slutsky's appointment as director of COE, she served as acting director of the Center for Practice and Technology Assessment at AHRQ. In 2005, Ms. Slutsky implemented a comparative-effectiveness research program that includes evidence synthesis, evidence gap analysis, evidence generation, and evidence translation and implementation. The Effective Health Care Program is authorized under Section 1013 of the Medicare Modernization Act. Ms. Slutsky oversees several outcomes and effectiveness research activities, including the Evidence-Based Practice Center program, Technology Assessment Program, extramural and intramural research portfolios concerning translating research into practice, pharmaceutical outcomes, and cost-effectiveness analyses, and the National Guideline, Quality Measures, and Health Care Innovations Exchange Clearinghouses. She is a member of the AcademyHealth Methods Council and a member of the Methods Committee of the Patient-Centered Outcomes Research Institute. Prior to becoming acting director of the Center for Practice and Technology Assessment, Ms. Slutsky served as project director of the U.S. Preventive Services Task Force, an internationally recognized panel of experts who make evidence-based recommendations on clinical preventive services. Ms. Slutsky received a BS (general science) at the University of Iowa and an MS in public health (health policy and administration) from the University of North Carolina at Chapel Hill and trained as a physician assistant at the University of Southern California.

Dylan Small, PhD, received a bachelor's degree in mathematics from Harvard University and a PhD degree in statistics from Stanford University. His dissertation was about instrumental variables regression, and his adviser Tze Leung Lai. Dr. Small started as an assistant professor in 2002 in the Department of Statistics of the Wharton School of the University of Pennsylvania. He was promoted to associate professor in 2008. Dr. Small's main areas of research interest are the following: design and analysis of experiments and observational studies for comparing treatments, policies, and programs; causal inference; measurement error; longitudinal data; and applications of statistics to improving health.

Harold Sox, MD, is a general internist and editor emeritus of the *Annals of Internal Medicine*. Dr. Sox spent most of his professional life at Stanford University and the Geisel School of Medicine at Dartmouth, the latter as chair of the department of medicine, and he is now associate director for faculty of The Dartmouth Institute for Health Policy and Clinical Practice. He chaired the U.S. Preventive Services Task Force, the Medicare Coverage Advisory Committee, and the Institute of Medicine's (IOM's) Committee to Set Priorities for Comparative Effectiveness Research. He was president of the American College of Physicians. He is a member of the IOM of the National Academy of Sciences. His books include *Medical Decision Making*, a standard textbook in this field.

Nicholas Tatonetti, PhD, joined the faculty at Columbia University in the department of biomedical informatics, Columbia Initiative in Systems Biology, and department of medicine in September 2012. His lab at Columbia is focused on expanding on his previous work at Stanford University in detecting drug effects and drug interactions from large-scale observational clinical data. Widely published in both clinical and bioinformatics, Dr. Tatonetti is passionate about the integration of hospital data (stored in electronic health records) and high-dimensional biological data (captured using next-generation sequencing, high-throughput screening, and other "omics" technologies). His lab develops the algorithms, techniques, and methods for analyzing enormous and diverse data by designing rigorous computational and mathematical approaches that address the fundamental challenges of observational analysis—bias and confounding. Foremost, they integrate medical observational with systems and chemical biology models to not only explain clinical observations but also to further our understanding of basic biology and human disease. Dr. Tatonetti has been featured as a rising star in the fields of computational biology and biomedical informatics by the *New York Times*, Genome Web, and Science Careers. His work as been picked up by the mainstream media and generated hundreds of news articles.

William S. Weintraub, MD, FACC, joined Christiana Care Health System in Delaware as cardiology section chief in 2005, after retiring from Emory University as professor emeritus of medicine and public health. Currently, Dr. Weintraub supervises the clinical, educational, research, and administrative activities of 20 full-time and 43 private-practice cardiologists as well as 15 cardiology fellows. He supervises busy interventional, noninvasive, and electrophysiology laboratories as well as an active heart failure service, spanning inpatient and outpatient care. Dr. Weintraub also holds appointments as professor of medicine at Jefferson University and professor of health sciences (adjunct) at the University of Delaware. Dr. Weintraub also leads the Christiana Care Center for Outcomes Research and is on the Research Committee and Coordinating Council of the Delaware Health Sciences Alliance. Dr. Weintraub was the first chairman of the National Cardiovascular Data Registry of the American College of Cardiology (ACC) and remains on the management board. Dr. Weintraub has also served on the American Heart Association (AHA) Database Executive Committee. He is the incoming chair of the AHA/ACC Task Force on Data Standards. Dr. Weintraub has also worked on multiple randomized clinical trials. These activities afforded him extensive experience participating in and leading multi-institutional research activities. Dr. Weintraub has specialized knowledge and skill in health status assessment and health care economics. He leads a $10 million innovation award from the Centers for Medicare & Medicaid Services to use advanced information technology and patient management to coordinate inpatient and outpatient care. In addition to extensive AHA and ACC committee activity, Dr. Weintraub has served on the ACC Board of Trustees and is currently president of the AHA

Great Rivers Affiliate. His multiple activities have focused on quality and outcomes of care, and he has deep experience in developing and assessing metrics to evaluate quality and outcomes.

John B. Wong, MD, FACP, is the chief of the Division of Clinical Decision Making, Informatics, and Telemedicine in the department of medicine of Tufts Medical Center and the Clinical and Translational Science Institute of the Tufts University School of Medicine and a practicing general internist. He is a past president of the Society for Medical Decision Making, the statistical editor in decision and cost-effectiveness analysis for the *Annals of Internal Medicine* at the American College of Physicians, co-director of the Tufts Evidence-Based Practice Center, and co-chair of the Methods Workgroup of the National Clinical Translational Sciences Award Strategic Goal Committee on Comparative Effectiveness Research. In addition to serving on study sections for the Agency for Healthcare Research and Quality and the National Institutes of Health, Dr. Wong has been a member of guideline committees for the American Association for the Study of Liver Disease Practice, the European League Against Rheumatism, OMERACT (Outcome Measures in Rheumatology), and the American College of Chest Physicians Antithrombotic Therapy. He has been the course director for evidence-based medicine at the Tufts University School of Medicine, the fellowship codirector for the National Library of Medicine–sponsored fellowship training program in medical informatics at Tufts Medical Center, and the medical informatics concentration leader for the Clinical Research Graduate Program of the Tufts University Sackler School of Biomedical Sciences. Dr. Wong's research focuses on the application of decision analysis to help patients, physicians, and policy makers choose among alternative tests, treatments, and policies and to promote rational evidence-based efficient and effective patient-centered care, reflecting individualized risk assessment and patient preferences. Dr. Wong received an MD from the University of Chicago and had postgraduate training in internal medicine at Tufts Medical Center.

Appendix B

Workshop Agenda

OBSERVATIONAL STUDIES IN A LEARNING HEALTH SYSTEM

❖

An Institute of Medicine Workshop
Sponsored by the Patient-Centered Outcomes Research Institute

❖

A Learning Health System Activity
IOM Roundtable on Value & Science-Driven Health Care

April 25–26, 2013

National Academy of Sciences
2101 Constitution Avenue, NW
Washington, DC

Meeting Objectives

1. Explore the role of observational studies (OSs) in the generation of evidence to guide clinical and health policy decisions, with a focus on individual patient care, in a learning health system;
2. Consider concepts of OS design and analysis, emerging statistical methods, use of OSs to supplement evidence from experimental methods, identifying treatment heterogeneity, and providing effectiveness estimates tailored for individual patients;
3. Engage colleagues from disciplines typically underrepresented in discussions of clinical evidence discussions; and
4. Identify strategies for accelerating progress in the appropriate use of OS for evidence generation.

Day 1: Thursday, April 25

8:00 am   Coffee and light breakfast available

8:30 am   **Welcome, introductions, and overview**
              Welcome, framing of the meeting, and agenda overview

              Welcome from the Institute of Medicine (IOM)
              Michael McGinnis, IOM

              Opening remarks and meeting overview
              Joe Selby, Patient-Centered Outcomes Research Institute
              Ralph Horwitz, GlaxoSmithKline

9:00 am   **Workshop stage setting**

              ➢ **Session format**
                  o **Workshop overview and stage setting**
                     Steve Goodman, Stanford University

                  Q&A and open discussion

              ➢ **Session questions:**
                  o How do observational studies contribute to building
                     valid evidence to support effective decision making by
                     patients and clinicians? When are their findings useful?
                     When are they not?
                  o What are the major challenges (study design,
                     methodological, data collection/management/
                     analysis, cultural, etc.) facing the field in the use of
                     observational study data for decision making? Please
                     include consideration of the following issues: bias,
                     methodological standards, publishing requirements.
                  o What can workshop participants expect from the
                     following sessions?

9:45 am   **Engaging the issue of bias**
              Moderator: *Michael Lauer*, National Heart, Lung, and
              Blood Institute

              ➢ **Session format**
                  o **Introduction to issue**
                     Sebastian Schneeweiss, Harvard University

o **Presentations:**
  ▪ Instrumental variables and their sensitivity to unobserved biases
    Dylan Small, University of Pennsylvania
  ▪ An empirical approach to measuring and calibrating for error in observational analyses
    Patrick Ryan, Johnson & Johnson

o **Respondents and panel discussion:**
  ▪ *John Wong*, Tufts University
  ▪ *Joel Greenhouse*, Carnegie Mellon University

Q&A and open discussion

➢ **Session questions:**
  o What are the major bias-related concerns with the use of observational study methods? What are the sources of bias?
  o How many of these concerns relate to methods and how many relate to the quality and availability of suitable data? What barriers have these concerns created for the use of the results of observational studies to drive decision making?
  o What are the most promising approaches to reduction of bias through the use of statistical methods? Through study design (e.g., dealing with issues of multiplicity)?
  o What are the circumstances under which administrative (claims) data can be used to assess treatment benefits? What data are needed from electronic health records to strengthen the value of administrative data?
  o What methods are best used to adjust for the changes in treatment and clinical conditions among patients followed longitudinally?
  o What are the implications of these promising approaches for the use of observational study methods moving forward?

11:30 am   Lunch

Participants will be asked to identify, along with the individuals at their table what they think the most critical questions are for patient centered research outcomes in the topics covered by the workshop. These topics will then be circulated to the moderators of the proceeding sessions.

12:30 pm   **Generalizing randomized controlled trial (RCT) results to broader populations**
Moderator: *Harold Sox*, Dartmouth College

➤ **Session format**
  o **Introduction to issue**
  Robert Califf, Duke

  o **Presentations:**
    ▪ Generalizing the right question
    Miguel Hernán, Harvard University
    ▪ Using observational studies to determine RCT generalizability
    Eloise Kaizar, The Ohio State University

  o **Respondents and panel discussion:**
    ▪ *William Weintraub*, Christiana Medical Center
    ▪ *Constantine Frangakis*, Johns Hopkins University

Q&A and open discussion

➤ **Session questions:**
  o What are the most cogent methodological and clinical considerations in the use of observational study methods to test the external validity of findings from RCTs?
  o How do data collection, management, and analysis approaches affect generalizability?
  o What are the generalizability questions of greatest interest? Or, where does the greatest doubt arise (age, concomitant illness, concomitant treatment)? What examples represent well-established differences?

o What statistical methods are needed to generalize RCT results?
o Are the standards for causal inference from OSs different when prior RCTs have been performed? How does statistical methodology vary in this case?
o What are the implications when treatment results for patients not included in the RCT differ from the overall results reported in the original RCT?
o What makes an observed difference in outcomes credible? Finding the effect shown in the RCT in the narrower population? Replication in more than one environment? The confidence interval of the result? The size of the effect in the RCT?
o Can subset analyses in the RCT, even if they are underpowered, be used to support or rebut the OS finding?

2:15 pm   **Break**

2:30 pm   **Detecting treatment effect heterogeneity**
Moderator: *Richard Platt*, Harvard Pilgrim Health Care Institute

➤ **Session format**
  o **Introduction to issue**
  David Kent, Tufts University

  o **Presentations:**
    ▪ Comparative effectiveness of coronary artery bypass grafting and percutaneous coronary intervention
    Mark Hlatky, Stanford University
    ▪ Identification of effect heterogeneity using instrumental variables
    Anirban Basu, University of Washington

  o **Respondents and panel discussion:**
    ▪ *Mary Charlson*, Cornell University
    ▪ *Mark Cullen*, Stanford University

Q&A and open discussion

➤ Session questions:
  ○ What is the potential for OSs in assessing treatment response heterogeneity and individual patient decision making?
  ○ What clinical and other data can be collected routinely to affect this potential?
  ○ How can longitudinal information on changes in treatment categories and clinical condition be used to assess variations in treatment responses and individual patient decision making?
    ▪ What are the statistical methods for time-varying changes in treatment (including cotherapies) and clinical condition?
  ○ What are the best methods to form distinctive patient subgroups in which to examine heterogeneity of the treatment response?
    ▪ What data elements are necessary to define these distinctive patient subgroups?
  ○ What are the best methods to assess heterogeneity in multidimensional outcomes?
  ○ How could further implementation of best practices in data collection, management, and analysis affect treatment response heterogeneity?
  ○ What is needed for information about treatment response heterogeneity to be validated and used in practice?

4:15 pm   **Summary and preview of next day**

4:45 pm   **Reception**

5:45 pm   **Adjourn**

Day 2: Friday, April 26

8:00 am   Coffee and light breakfast available

8:30 am   **Welcome, brief agenda overview, and summary of previous day**
           Welcome, framing of the meeting, and agenda overview

9:00 am   **Predicting individual responses**
                 Moderator: *Ralph Horwitz*, GlaxoSmithKline

                 ➢ **Session format**
                     ○ **Introduction to issue**
                     Burton Singer, University of Florida

                     ○ **Presentations:**
                         ▪ Data-driven prediction models
                           Nicholas Tatonetti, Columbia University
                         ▪ Individual prediction
                           Michael Kattan, Cleveland Clinic

                     ○ **Respondents and panel discussion:**
                         ▪ *Peter Bach*, Sloan Kettering
                         ▪ *Mitchell Gail*, National Cancer Institute

                     Q&A and open discussion

                 ➢ **Session questions:**
                     ○ How can patient-level observational data be used to create predictive models of the treatment response in individual patients? What statistical methodologies are needed?
                     ○ How can predictive analytic methods be used to study the interactions of treatment with multiple patient characteristics?
                     ○ How should the clinical history (longitudinal information) for a given patient be utilized in the creation of rules to predict the response of that patient to one or more candidate treatment regimens?
                     ○ What are effective methodologies for producing prediction rules to guide the management of an individual patient on the basis of their comparability to the results of RCTs, OSs, and archived patient records?
                     ○ How can we blend predictive models, which can predict impact of treatment choices, and causal modeling, that compare predictions under different treatments?

10:45 am   **Break**

11:00 am   **Conclusions and strategies going forward**
Panel members will be charged with highlighting very
specific next steps laid out in the course of workshop
presentations and discussions or suggesting some of their
own.

> ➢ **Panel:**
>   o *Cynthia D. Mulrow*, University of Texas
>   o *Jean R. Slutsky*, Agency for Healthcare Research and
>   Quality
>   o *Steven N. Goodman*, Stanford University

> ➢ **Session questions:**
>   o What are the major themes and conclusions from the
>   workshop's presentations and discussions?
>   o How can these themes be translated into actionable
>   strategies with designated stakeholders?
>   o What are the critical next steps in terms of advancing
>   analytic methods?
>   o What are the critical next steps in developing
>   databases that will generate evidence to guide clinical
>   decision making?
>   o What are critical next steps in disseminating
>   information on new methods to increase their
>   appropriate use?

12:15 pm   **Summary and next steps**

Comments from the Chairs
Joe Selby, Patient-Centered Outcomes Research Institute
Ralph Horwitz, GlaxoSmithKline

Comments and thanks from the IOM
Michael McGinnis, IOM

12:45 pm   **Adjourn**

Planning Committee

Co-Chairs

Ralph I. Horwitz, GlaxoSmithKline
Joe V. Selby, Patient-Centered Outcomes Research Institute

Members

Anirban Basu, University of Washington
Troyen A. Brennan, CVS/Caremark
Steven N. Goodman, Stanford University
Louis B. Jacques, Centers for Medicare & Medicaid Services
Jerome P. Kassirer, Tufts University School of Medicine
Michael S. Lauer, National Heart, Lung, and Blood Institute
David Madigan, Columbia University
Sharon-Lise T. Normand, Harvard University
Richard Platt, Harvard Pilgrim Health Care Institute
Burton H. Singer, University of Florida
Jean R. Slutsky, Agency for Healthcare Research and Quality
Robert Temple, U.S. Food and Drug Administration

Staff Officer

Claudia Grossmann
cgrossmann@nas.edu
202.334.3867

Appendix C

Workshop Participants

Jill Abell, PhD, MPH
Senior Director, Clinical
  Effectiveness and Safety
GlaxoSmithKline

Naomi Aronson
Executive Director
Blue Cross Blue Shield

Peter Bach, MD, MAPP
Attending Physician
Department of Epidemiology &
  Biostatistics
Memorial Sloan-Kettering Cancer
  Center

Anirban Basu, MS, PhD
Associate Professor and Director
Program in Health Economics and
  Outcomes Methodology
University of Washington

Lawrence Becker
Director, Benefits
Xerox Corporation

Marc L. Berger, MD
Vice President, Real World Data
  and Analytics
Pfizer Inc.

Robert M. Califf, MD
Vice Chancellor for Clinical
  Research
Duke University Medical Center

Mary E. Charlson, MD
Chief, Clinical Epidemiology and
  Evaluative Sciences Research
Weill Cornell Medical College

Jennifer B. Christian, PharmD,
  MPH, PhD
Senior Director, Clinical
  Effectiveness and Safety
GlaxoSmithKline

Mark R. Cullen, MD
Professor of Medicine
Stanford University School of
  Medicine

Steven R. Cummings, MD, FACP
Professor Emeritus, Department of
   Medicine
University of California, San
   Francisco

Robert W. Dubois, MD, PhD
Chief Science Officer
National Pharmaceutical Council

Rachael L. Fleurence, PhD
Acting Director, Accelerating
   PCORI Methods Program
PCORI

Dean Follmann, PhD
Branch Chief-Associate Director
   for Biostatistics
National Institutes of Health

Constantine Frangakis, PhD
Professor, Department of
   Biostatistics
Johns Hopkins Bloomberg School
   of Public Health

Mitchell H. Gail, MD, PhD
Senior Investigator
National Cancer Institute

Kathleen R. Gans-Brangs, PhD
Senior Director, Medical Affairs
AstraZeneca

Steven N. Goodman, MD, PhD
Associate Dean for Clinical and
   Translational Research
Stanford University School of
   Medicine

Sheldon Greenfield, MD
Executive Co-Director, Health
   Policy Research Institute
University of California, Irvine

Joel B. Greenhouse, PhD
Professor of Statistics
Carnegie Mellon University

Sean Hennessy, PharmD, PhD
Associate Professor of
   Epidemiology
University of Pennsylvania

Miguel Hernán, MD, DrPH, ScM,
   MPH
Professor of Epidemiology
Harvard University

Mark A. Hlatky, MD
Professor, Stanford Health Policy
   Fellow
Department of Health Research
   and Policy
Stanford University

Ralph I. Horwitz, M.D.
Senior Vice President, Clinical
   Science Evaluation
GlaxoSmithKline

Gail Hunt
President and Chief Executive
   Officer
National Alliance for Caregiving

Robert Jesse, MD, PhD
Principal Deputy Under Secretary
   for Health
Department of Veterans Affairs

Eloise E. Kaizar, PhD
Associate Professor
Department of Statistics
The Ohio State University

Jerome P. Kassirer, MD
Distinguished Professor
Tufts University School of
    Medicine

Michael Kattan, PhD
Quantitative Health Sciences
    Department Chair
Cleveland Clinic

David M. Kent, MD, MSc
Director, Clinical and Translational
    Science Program
Tufts University Sackler School of
    Graduate Biomedical Sciences

Michael S. Lauer, MD, FACC,
    FAHA
Director, Division of
    Cardiovascular Sciences
National Heart, Lung, and Blood
    Institute

J. Michael McGinnis, MD, MPP,
    MA
Senior Scholar
Institute of Medicine

David O. Meltzer, PhD
Associate Professor
University of Chicago

Nancy E. Miller, PhD
Senior Science Policy Analyst
Office of Science Policy
National Institutes of Health

Sally Morton, PhD
Professor and Chair, Department of
    Biostatistics
Graduate School of Public Health
University of Pittsburgh

Cynthia D. Mulrow, MD, MSc
Senior Deputy Editor
Annals of Internal Medicine

Robin Newhouse
Chair and Associate Professor
University of Maryland School of
    Nursing

Perry D. Nisen, MD, PhD
SVP, Science and Innovation
GlaxoSmithKline

Richard Platt, MD, MS
Chair, Ambulatory Care and
    Prevention
Chair, Population Medicine
Harvard University

James Robins, MD
Mitchell L. and Robin
    LaFoley Dong Professor of
    Epidemiology
Harvard University

Patrick Ryan, PhD
Head of Epidemiology Analytics
Janssen Research and Development

Nancy Santanello, MD, MS
Vice President, Epidemiology
Merck & Co.

Richard L. Schilsky, MD, FASCO
Chief Medical Officer
American Society of Clinical
    Oncology

Sebastian Schneeweiss, MD
Associate Professor, Epidemiology
Division of Pharmacoepidemiology
    and Pharmacoeconomics
Brigham and Women's Hospital

J. Sanford Schwartz, MD
Leon Hess Professor in Internal
    Medicine
University of Pennsylvania School
    of Medicine

Jodi Segal, MD, MPH
Director, Pharmacoepidemiology
    Program
The John Hopkins Medical
    Institutions

Joe V. Selby, MD, MPH
Executive Director
PCORI

Burton H. Singer, PhD, MS
Professor, Emerging Pathogens
    Institute
University of Florida

Jean Slutsky, PA, MS
Director, Center for Outcomes and
    Evidence
Agency for Healthcare Research
    and Quality

Dylan Small, PhD
Associate Professor of Statistics
University of Pennsylvania

Harold C. Sox, MD
Professor of Medicine
Dartmouth Geisel School of
    Medicine

Elizabeth A. Stuart
Associate Professor, Department of
    Biostatistics
Johns Hopkins Bloomberg School
    of Public Health

Nicholas Tatonetti, PhD
Assistant Professor of Biomedical
    Informatics
Columbia University

Robert Temple, MD
Deputy Center Director for Clinical
    Science
U.S. Food and Drug
    Administration

William S. Weintraub, MD, FACC
John H. Ammon Chair of
    Cardiology
Christiana Care Health Services

Harlan Weisman
Managing Director
And-One Consulting, LLC

John B. Wong, MD
Professor of Medicine
Tufts University Sackler School of
    Graduate Biomedical Sciences